REMEMBERING ANN

With best wishes

J M

'I can testify with certainty that there are significant riverbeds of progress and joy that wind through my soul as a result of Ann Goldingay.'   **Erika Haub**

'Ann, you are helpless, vulnerable and fragile. By your very presence, you bring out those fears in me. And I realize that my world really isn't that safe and I am not as much in control as I think I am or as I want to be. ... You teach me that to be human is to live in a world that is neither perfect nor safe. You invite me to trust God and live my life in complete dependence on Him, in whom we live, move, and have our being.'   **Sol Nuñez**

And When Did You Last See Ann?

Was it the last time she was able to raise her eyebrow?
Was it the last time she smiled?
Was it the last time she swallowed?
Was it the last time she laughed?
Was it the last time she said 'John'?
Was it the last time she cried?
Was it the last time she transferred to a pew in church?
Was it the last time she signed her name?
...   **John Goldingay**

REMEMBERING ANN

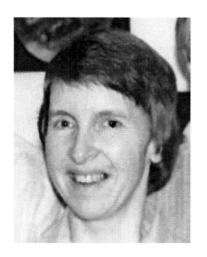

by
John Goldingay

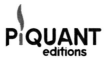

P**i**QUANT
editions

First published in Great Britain by Piquant in 2011
PO Box 83, Carlisle, CA3 9GR, UK
www.piquanteditions.com

ISBN 978-1-903689-75-2

British Library Cataloguing in Publication Data

Goldingay, John.
  Remembering Ann.
  1. Goldingay, John--Marriage. 2. Goldingay, Ann.
  3. Goldingay, Ann--Marriage. 4. Goldingay, Ann--Health.
  5. Multiple sclerosis--Patients--Biography. 6. Multiple
  sclerosis--Patients--Family relationships.
  I. Title
  362.1'96834'0092-dc22

Cover design by Projectluz
Cover photographs © John Goldingay
Typesetting by To a Tee

CONTENTS

PREFACE

On a bright English April morning I first met her—a bright, pretty, bushy-tailed, wide-eyed nineteen-year-old girl at a student conference. On a bright Californian June morning forty-six years later, I took her to Urgent Care because she wasn't breathing very well, and a few hours later she stopped breathing at all. For the months that have since passed, I have been missing her, and watching myself missing her, and wondering about the meaning of my life without her.

That story outline has been replicated and filled out millions of times in the lives of millions of couples. While it's special to me because it's mine, it's just an ordinary story. Yet I have discovered that it is special to other people. This arises out of the fact that for forty-three of those years Ann lived with an illness that eventually left her not only wheelchair-bound but unable to swallow or speak. Somehow the way she handled that experience had a profound effect on people (not to say me). Here are three comments from the days after her death:

> *'Ann was a quiet (mainly!) yet somewhat revolutionary presence in St John's Theological College. I remember coming for interview and seeing the wheelchair lift on the stairs and immediately thinking "there's more to this place*

than the headlines," long before the church had thought very much about disability. I remember her delight at certain things and the infectiousness of her laughter and her smile. And I remember seeing you and her together and watching the impact of life at St John's and of Ann's illness on you and the holding of that within Christian community in creative as well as tough ways. Ann for me was one of the people who kept the place grounded; when it became most hothouse-like, seeing Ann at chapel or in meals helped me to hold things in proportion.'

'It can be the most unlikely person who impacts us the most deeply. It was not surprising that, as a student at Fuller Seminary, I would find myself challenged and provoked by an Old Testament professor named John Goldingay. What I did not expect was to have my life changed by the mostly silent woman who sat in a wheelchair. ... I can testify with certainty that there are significant riverbeds of progress and joy that wind through my soul as a result of Ann Goldingay.'

'I love this sentence, "But I can testify with certainty that there are significant riverbeds of progress and joy that wind through my soul as a result of Ann Goldingay." Add two more of us to the number. ... We are forever grateful that she paid the price of her discipleship because she stands tall in a very small group of fellow believers who have worked for our comfort and edification, instead of harm. Her direct contribution to our ministry is, without a doubt, one of the greatest gifts we have ever received.'

(I should explain for UK readers that a seminary is a theological college, and for US readers that a theological college is a seminary.)

The chapters that follow tell Ann's story, pass on some of the comments people have made on her significance for them, and reflect on what grieving her has been like.   *John Goldingay*

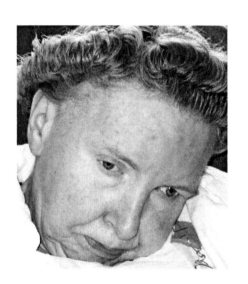

— I —

Your Story

Ann had multiple sclerosis. Being wheelchair bound as she was for the last twelve years of life makes a person susceptible to pneumonia. She had pneumonia four or five times. Each time experts assured me it would be the end of her, though apparently she and/or God had other ideas. On one of those occasions when she came home from hospital on 'hospice care' (that is, we would have some support at home for what was assumed would be a short period so that she could die at home) the hospice people provided me with various useful resources, one of which encouraged a married couple to spend time talking over their life during what was expected to be their last weeks or months. Because Ann couldn't speak, we couldn't do precisely this, and because I am by nature a writer, what I began to do was write our story. I think I may have done this for my sake but also so I could read it to Ann. I didn't keep going at it for very long, partly because she as usual declined to die and we resumed our usual unusual life, but after she died I took it up again, and I imagine reading it to her as she lies in her resting place waiting for resurrection day. I have rewritten it a little to provide the background information that wasn't needed when it was meant only for us, but I have left it in the form of address to her.

Beginnings

You and I met at a Christian student conference at Swanwick in Derbyshire in England in April 1963. The single *Please Please Me* had just been number one; the album *Please Please Me* was about to be number one. You were a medical student in London; I was a theology student at Oxford. We happened to sit next to each other one morning at breakfast. You were probably with your friend Ann Pretty, eventually your bridesmaid, and I may have been with my friend John Alexander. I was wearing my name badge upside down and I think you asked me why (it's just the kind of thing I do). You may have been wearing pink. We discussed the fact that the boiled eggs were hard on the inside and soft on the outside, and we wondered how that happened. The four of us spent a chunk of time together over the week. I can't remember if I was looking for someone; I think probably not, as I was going out with someone else, though I knew this relationship wasn't the one that was going to be forever. I think you were going out with someone else in London. We didn't exchange addresses or anything.

The next year we went back to Swanwick, each wondering if the other would be there. I had broken off with the other girl just beforehand, but you were still going out with someone. Again we spent a lot of time together. I don't remember if Ann Pretty and John Alexander were there but my lifelong friend Roger Finney was, and he still remembers you as 'the lovely and lively teenager at Swanwick'. The last night, we sat on the purple sofa in the entrance hall in front of the coal fire and ended up kissing and embracing till 2 a.m., in that rather public place. In future years we often went back to Swanwick and paid our respects to the sofa, and we were sorry that in due course it wore out and had to be replaced.

After Swanwick we both went home for the rest of the Easter break; I then returned to Oxford before you returned to London. We must have written to each other, because I knew you were coming back to London by train on a certain Sunday and I went to London to meet you off the train. You knew I might be coming and you also knew that the other guy might be coming, so you worried over this with Ann Pretty all the way to London. But only I showed up, so I won.

I then went back to Oxford for my last term and final exams (comps, in US-speak). I came to see you in London a couple of times, I think, and you came to Oxford once. Then, when exam week arrived, you sent me a red rose by Interflora each day (you got a special deal because the florist took pity on you in your poverty as a student). On the Saturday in the middle of the week you showed up unannounced and met me after the exam. I still remember coming out of the exam room and seeing you there. You came again for the May Ball a couple of weeks later. We stayed up all night (well, we had a nap in a borrowed room in the early hours) then went boating at dawn. After the end of term I went to Torquay in the southwest of England to work as a waiter in a hotel, but I had to go back to Oxford for my oral exam (defense, in US-speak), and as a result of a confusion had an extra day off, and consequently had time to hitchhike to London afterwards to see you.

I was due to go to Bristol for ordination training in October 1964. Because you were in London, it now seemed more sensible to go to the London College of Divinity and I consulted a mentor about that, Alec Motyer, the Vice-Principal in Bristol. Not surprisingly, he thought I should stick with the original decision to go to Bristol. While I was there, you and I wrote to each other alternate days, I think; I often wrote during lectures. Once or twice a term I would go to London to see you. The theological college rules did not allow me to be away overnight, so I would get the 3.45 a.m. train to London on a Sunday and return on the 11.50 p.m. one, which got back at 3.15 a.m on Monday morning. You were living near Marble Arch; after spending the day with you, I would walk to Paddington to get the train, and more than once almost missed it. I remember a time when we had an Indian meal in Edgware Road at the end of one of those fabulous Sunday evenings. I remember how full of energy you were. I remember some occasion when you were skipping along a passage at your hall of residence in a slight summer dress, then dancing around your room, and I was so aware of your lively physicality. You also came to Bristol from time to time, and I remember going to see the first James Bond film on a dark rainy evening, and on another occasion picnicking in a field on a bright summer day.

Diagnosis

You were a top student at your medical school and also about now you became lady vice-president of the London University Christian Fellowship; there was a glass ceiling for women (I think there probably still is), so this was as high as a woman could get. In spring 1965 you were staying temporarily in someone's apartment in Hampstead, overlooking a railway line, and we spent a chunk of the Easter break there. You were also working, dissecting in the Anatomy Department of your medical school for demonstration purposes. You developed a great enthusiasm for anatomy; you could get ecstatic about *Gray's Anatomy* in the days before it was a TV programme. You took some photos of the body you were dissecting, and the pharmacist who developed them thought about calling the police because he wondered if you were a murderer. You subsequently moved into a four-girl apartment off Abbey Road where the Beatles did their recording, and I stayed there several times over the next year, sleeping on the sofa in the lounge (or did I sleep in your bed while you slept on the sofa?). Sometimes I slept in the apartment belonging to the boyfriend of one of the other girls, because your parents disapproved of my staying in the apartment. We had tortuous discussions about whether we ought to do what they said even though we thought there was nothing wrong with me staying there and we weren't actually sleeping together.

In summer 1965 I again worked in Torquay but also had some time staying with you and some time on a church placement in Walthamstow in East London. I think it was that December we saw the Beatles at the Hammersmith Odeon, though you were not pleased that the young girls were screaming so loudly that you couldn't hear John and Paul. At Christmas I came to Stockton to meet your parents. We knew we were in love with each other but we felt we needed to have a sense of whether it was God's will for us to marry. On the bus on the way somewhere on New Year's Eve you told me you thought God was saying 'Yes', and I was prepared to go with that, though I had no independent sense of God saying this. I twisted a strand of thin gold Christmas decoration round your finger. You kept that for years; I think it is still in your jewellery box.

At Easter 1966 I came to stay with you for a day or two and you had developed a limp. I must have arrived on a Sunday because I remember we were walking to the subway to get to church when I could see this limp and you told me that you thought you had Disseminated Sclerosis, as it was then known. You explained what this meant. That week you went to your own hospital and, after rolling their eyes at the way medical students imagine they have all the worst illnesses, they confirmed your self-diagnosis. The following Sunday I hitchhiked back from Bristol to London to see you. It was a lovely sunny spring day and I got a lift all the way from Bristol to London in a sports car. I felt full of joy from God.

You went into hospital for two weeks while they gave you steroid injections. You got upset because these made you put on weight and come out in spots, but the shots sorted out the symptoms. I came to see you again when you were due to leave hospital. We had both felt very close to God as we went through this crisis. Then as we left the hospital we had an argument about whether we should go home on the bus or on the tube. It was like a bubble bursting.

In the summer of 1966 after I finished at theological college I went to Torquay once more but also stayed with you for some weeks. I think we got engaged that summer. We had waited because your parents were against it. They didn't like me, and they didn't wish to lose their daughter, but it seemed that waiting longer wasn't going to make any difference, and you wanted an engagement ring on my finger before I arrived in the parish. I remember us going to a jeweller's at Kings Cross where we chose rings together. The sun was shining. We couldn't afford much. We chose a zircon for you, a lovely pale blue colour, which I think cost £23 ($40), and a plain signet ring for me; I can't remember the cost.

In September I was ordained and began work at Christ Church in North Finchley, London, moving into the apartment next to the church. During that year I would come down to Hampstead to see you on Tuesdays, my day off, and you would come up to Christ Church on Sundays. The apartment was very public. We would resort to the corridor between the living room and the kitchen for kissing and cuddling, and once burned a pan of rice when we got too preoccupied.

Marriage

The apartment was officially a single man's apartment, a bed-sit with a kitchen and bathroom, but there was another room at the front of the house (I think it was used for parish meetings), and the church agreed that it could become part of the apartment. I had to get the bishop's permission to get married, but he was sympathetic, not least because his son was a medical student and he knew a medical student's life was complicated. We arranged to get married on your mother's birthday, hoping that this might encourage relationships. It didn't.

In April 1967, a few months before the wedding date, you had another relapse of the MS, this time affecting your eyes, but the drug again did the trick. I think it was on this occasion that a nurse said you had no business getting married and having children when you had this disease. She was wrong, wasn't she?

Over the early summer you made new curtains for the apartment, cutting them out on a table tennis table in a hospital residence. We bought second-hand furniture (a bed, a wardrobe, and a dressing table) from a woman in the congregation. You said you wouldn't go through with the wedding unless I acquired a fridge and a washer-drier. We borrowed a hatchback from a couple in the congregation to move your stuff, but I couldn't quite close the back doors when everything was in, and as we waited at traffic lights on a hill, your medical journals started sliding out the back onto the road. I got measured up for a suit for the only time in my life; when we next met, you asked me what the suit was like, and I said 'blue, green, and red stripes', which it is, though they are very discrete stripes, but it made you panic for a moment.

We married on the late summer holiday Monday, 28 August 1967. For our honeymoon, the plan had been to go to a cottage in Devon belonging to the mother of a friend of yours, but there had been a misunderstanding and you discovered on the Thursday before the wedding that the cottage was not available. Having made that discovery, you went off to Stockton to get ready for the wedding. That evening I mentioned this as a prayer topic to a member of the church with whom I was having dinner. Next day his sister called to offer a cottage at the very centre of Wales (on the north-south axis) and on the very east (on the east-west axis); actually it was in England, but Wales was at the bottom of the garden.

On the Sunday I took part in the morning service in Finchley then drove up to Stockton, again in the borrowed hatchback. I stayed with your Auntie Olive so that I didn't see you on the morning of the wedding even when I had to drop by your house to get something. She made me bacon and egg for breakfast and we joked about the prisoner's last meal before the execution. I set up the tape recording for the service and switched it on just before you arrived looking lovely in your white dress. My rector, Harold Parks, married us. It was very important to your parents that he should say both your Christian names, but unfortunately he forgot your second name (though he remembered mine). At the reception we had Brussels sprouts (among other things). Afterwards we changed into our going-away things—or rather you did, because I was keeping my suit on. You looked fabulous in a short-skirted pink outfit, and a hat, I think. I was afraid people would sabotage the car or otherwise play tricks on us, in accordance with British wedding customs, so we left the reception in another car in order to transfer a little way away. Anxious about the tricks, I shut the car door on your coat, and you got annoyed with me; it was our first marital tiff. We drove off in the gloom, rain, and traffic jams of an end-of-holiday evening, and I diverted off the A1 onto the A61 to drive through Leeds and Sheffield as it got dark. We were thus a bit late getting to the hotel in Dovedale, not far from Swanwick where we met, but it was okay. We made love for the first time, and it seemed to be satisfactory for both of us, unless you were faking; but you've never been much of a faker.

We didn't sleep very long; we were up at 6 a.m. looking out of the window at the bright sunshine and the cows grazing on the hills across the dale. After breakfast we walked down Dovedale along the river and crossed the river by the stepping stones. That is where I said I would scatter your ashes, and where I will ask Steven and Mark to scatter mine. You were wearing a little cotton dress, white with a flowery pattern. It was a lovely morning.

We then drove to Wales. Unfortunately it rained for the week, as it often does there (it was some years before I managed to get you back to Wales). So we did a lot of driving all round the northern half of the country. In the rain I nearly totalled the car one day. At the pottery at Portmeirion we bought the two large rich blue cups that now sit on the glass shelves in our apartment (the cups used to have saucers, but those got broken).

After a week you declared that this was enough of this rainy place and please could we now go to Devon as arranged. We had bed and breakfast near Exeter and went to see a film for the first time as a married couple. The next day we drove on, not sure where we were going to stay. We dropped in at the hotel in Torquay where I used to work, coffee became a free lunch, and then they invited us to stay the week for free in a spare single room adapted a bit for us.

Motherhood

At the end of September 1967 I was ordained as a priest and the next day we left at 5 p.m. to drive to Stockton in a rental car for your cousin's wedding, and to bring your dad back to London for a hip operation. I fell asleep on the way back and we had a providential escape from this story coming to an end that day.

Two months later you were pregnant, despite the fact that you were on the contraceptive pill. When you were throwing up, at first we thought you had flu, but eventually you had a pregnancy test. The following Friday the *British Medical Journal* printed an article declaring that the pill you were on was not as effective as some others; we could confirm that.

Because of the implications for your studies, your parents couldn't have been more furious if we had been unmarried. They saw the entire fault as mine for not looking after birth control in a more traditional fashion. More significantly, your neurologist, P.K. Thomas, whom you loved, was concerned because of the stress associated with pregnancy for someone with MS, and he wanted you to have an abortion. We asked for a second opinion and went to see a Dr P.C. Gautier-Smith (who I have discovered also writes crime stories, unless there are two people with that distinctive name). His comments, as I remember them (though you could not remember this) included the observation that he quite believed from the notes that you had MS, but he could not find any evidence of it in your body. That was a kind of sign. You continued with the pregnancy, and there is Steven, now grown up and married with children of his own.

In the event, the pregnancy was fairly straightforward. During the early months you passed one set of medical finals. In June we had a lovely holiday in a cliff-top cottage overlooking the sea in Cornwall, when the number one record was *I Say a Little Prayer for You* and the number two was *This Guy's in Love with You*, both of which were true. I have photos of you sporting yourself on the cliff-top seven-months-gone in a little shirt and panties, drinking milk straight from a bottle.

In the later weeks of the pregnancy you went into hospital because you had high blood pressure. In the early hours of 28 August your Professor of Obstetrics called to tell me to get down to the hospital if I was to see the action. It was not usual in those days for husbands to be present when a baby was born, but you wanted me there so I would stop saying I didn't believe what they said about how it worked. We were expecting a girl, code-named Freda, because everyone else we knew was having boys (again, in those days there were no ultrasounds that meant people could know the baby's sex). The Professor's first words were, 'It's Fred not Freda.' After a few days you were allowed home with Steven. Because he had long fingernails he needed mitts to prevent him scratching himself, and we stopped on the Holloway Road for you to go to a baby store. The panic I felt at being left alone with the baby is a more vivid memory than the birth.

For reasons I only half-understood, you had to take two sets of medical finals, covering the same syllabus for different examining bodies (it now seems quite uncivilized). You took the second set a few months after Steven's birth. Other than that, you didn't have work obligations until the following summer. I was then due to move on from the church where I was working. I had been asked to consider theological college teaching and had decided to do a further degree in that connection, so we moved onto the campus at Oak Hill Theological College nearby, where I did some teaching to pay the rent while also studying in London. For roughly the same year you did residences at your medical school's hospitals in London. We bought a carpet square for the house we were moving into and I crashed the car on the way home with the carpet in the back of the hatchback (a different one) and you sitting in the front with Steven on your lap (there were no seat belts for anyone in those days); rather amazingly, no one was hurt.

We found a young woman called Mary as a live-in nanny for Steven, Monday to Friday; I think you came home alternate nights and alternate weekends. When you were on duty at the weekend I would take Steven down to the hospital and you would bath him and get him ready for bed there, before I brought him home to sleep. I have a vivid memory of our going out one winter evening to see *Butch Cassidy and the Sundance Kid*. As we walked through the rainy parking lot, you asked me 'What kind of film is it?' 'I think it's a kind-of Western.' You stopped dead. 'I'm not going to see a Western!' 'I think it's a different sort of Western,' I said, defensively. It became one of your all-time favourite films. But in principle you were never very keen on what you would call 'waste-of-time films', ones with no deep treatment of relationships or deep message about something.

Moving from London

The end of your residences year in the summer of 1970 more or less coincided with the end of my year of further study, so we could be pretty open about where we went next. You had once wanted to be a surgeon, but because of the illness you had been advised to think in terms of a physically less-demanding specialty. Ever since working as a volunteer in some psychiatric setting when you were still at high school you had also been attracted to psychiatry, so I think your game plan was that wherever we moved, you would hope to have another baby and do some part-time work in primary care medicine for a while, then get into a postgraduate programme in psychiatry; and that is what you managed.

When I was offered a post a St John's Theological College in Nottingham, a hundred miles north of London and between the homes of our two sets of parents, you were willing for me to accept it, though you were nervous about leaving London; all your professional networks were there. I have two memories of our first Sunday in Nottingham. When we were trying to get our two-year-old ready for church, a slightly dishevelled figure appeared at the back door whom you greeted without enthusiasm not realizing that it was my boss coming to give us a word of welcome. He was one of the best-known evangelical figures in England and widely recognized, but not by you. Then at church the lay preacher was a local physician, Alan Murphy, who spoke about the way the human birth process helps us understand spiritual birth. Afterwards you went to talk to him and he offered you just the sort of job you wanted, part-time work in general practice as a primary care physician.

The next bit of your life plan was to have that other baby, and quick. Fulfilling this aim did require my cooperation. I learned more than I needed to know about how to improve the chances of conception, which involved contortions in bed that I won't detail; I remember having an amused and slightly hurt sense that I was just an adjunct to this project rather than being involved in an adventure in lovemaking. I guess this is an equivalent to (or an obverse of) what women often feel about sex. It worked, though, and you were soon pregnant (nowadays the verb 'be pregnant' has become gender-inclusive, but I have not been able to make that transfer of usage). But you had a miscarriage on the day after Christmas Day (what British people call Boxing Day, after the fact that this was the day alms boxes used to be opened and gifts given to the needy). We were at your parents' home and a few days later we were all watching a New Year review programme on TV that included shots of babies in some connection, and you were in tears on the sofa. That was when I learned that having a miscarriage was a deeper experience than I realized.

You soon resumed inviting me to service you and indulging in your contortions and you were soon pregnant again. Thinking about it now I wonder if you were some kind of super-fertile woman, since you got pregnant at the drop of a hat (without the drop of a hat, the first time). In recent years we have had many student friends who have found it hard to get pregnant (I am on the verge of using that verb gender-inclusively). They do tend to be older than we were, though now I come to think about it you were twenty-seven. (You were twenty-four when Steven was born, and were offended that the medical staff called you an 'elderly primigravida', someone rather old to be pregnant for the first time; I think they may have been joking, but I didn't realize it.)

The pregnancy was uneventful and you went into labour on New Year's Eve. I thought we might make the newspapers for having the first baby of 1972, but the labour was very quick and we didn't even have the last of 1971. Just after 7 p.m. you were lying on a gurney in the hospital corridor, waiting to be moved into a room. You told the nurses the baby was coming and they urged you to wait till they had the room ready. 'I can't wait!' you protested, but you did have Mark in the room rather than in the corridor. Having hung around for a bit I went home, I guess partly to collect Steven from wherever we had left him. I put him to bed and thought about the fact that we had been invited to a New Year's party two doors away, so I dropped by to tell people and wet the baby's head, as they say in the northeast (that is, have a drink in its honour) and to welcome the New Year. While I was out, you called and got no answer and were not impressed when I later confessed that I was off partying in your absence and leaving Steven in the house on his own (which was also illegal).

Getting Back to Work

After Mark was born, the way you initially found your way back into medicine was by doing birth control clinics in the evening once a week. I got left with both children. Mark was a few months old and would invariably start crying before you went out and continue to do so much of the time you were out. You told me that this might be partly because he had been able to sense your anxiety in getting ready to go out and leave him with his stupid theologian father, but also because he had 'six month colic'. I thought you told me it was because his insides were not yet fully formed, though I did not find this when I Googled the expression just now to make sure I had it right. I did find the information that 'living with an infant suffering from colic can really drive a parent to their wits' end. You may feel incompetent, depressed, or downright angry when all attempts to stop your baby's crying seem useless.' Too right! Living with it for a couple of hours could do that!

In due course you also went back to being a part-time primary care physician and started especially seeing patients who needed something more like counselling or psychotherapy, which encouraged the development of a sense that you wanted to specialize in this area. At this point 'coincidence' and the great Alan Murphy again intervened. His next-door neighbour was none other than the professor of Psychiatry in the recently-established Medical School in Nottingham. They were about to begin postgraduate training in psychiatry, a four-year programme that could be undertaken part-time over eight years. So Alan had a conversation with the professor over the back garden fence and you joined the first cohort on that programme in September 1973.

For the summer we stayed in Israel, where I undertook a locum at the Anglican congregation in Tel Aviv and did some archeology, and we spent time soaking up the land. Among my favourite photos are ones of you changing Mark's diaper on the tailgate of a station wagon and of you riding a camel near Jericho, looking rather precarious but laughing, with your short dress riding practically up to your thighs. In the few days after our return from Israel we moved from a house off the campus into one on the campus, Steven started at 'proper' school, and you started the programme in psychiatry. You then generally spent the mornings at the hospital where the programme was based, while Mark was looked after by our next-door neighbour, Eileen (on the way to becoming wife of the Archbishop of Canterbury, but none of us dreamed that); her youngest was within a few weeks of being the same age as Mark. For some while Mark, who was not yet two, would cry every morning when you set off for work, which was hard. For him, there were so many changes all at once; we had all been together through the summer, then suddenly we moved house, Steven went to school, I went back to work, and you went off to the hospital.

Over the next eight years you completed the programme according to the schedule and we lived a fairly uneventful and busy life focused on work and home (I often tell people I know nothing of the music between 1969 and 1984 because we were busy bringing up children). The illness didn't have much effect, though you would sometimes run out of energy. I remember us once taking a long Sunday walk on a crisp January afternoon and you reaching a point when you couldn't walk any further. I was scared. We were half a mile from a road, but we sat on a bench for half an hour and you recovered strength.

You also did have occasional proper relapses of the illness. The two recurrent symptoms were your eyes going out of focus and your having difficulty walking. On one such occasion we were about to go on holiday, so Alan showed me how to give you injections of the drug. Doing so was scary for me, but you took it in your stride ('Stick it in *there*!). On another occasion Alan was on holiday and his stand-in decided to try a different form of the drug, which sent you manic. You would try to do far too much and not be able to complete anything, and you would wake up with the sun early in the morning; it was May and sunrise was about 5 a.m. For several consecutive days, when you awoke you would have a message from God in your head. These were obviously psychotic delusions. Except that when you then read the Bible and the Bible

Reading notes that you used, you would find the word from God confirmed in what you read there.

I have many great photos from this period that confirm the reminiscences of people, that you continued to be lively, bright, and smiling.

Psychiatry

In 1981 you passed the final exams that qualified you to become a Member of the Royal College of Psychiatrists. Taking them involved an odd experience that with hindsight hinted at a change in the effect of the illness on you. It was only forty miles to the exam location in Birmingham but you didn't want to drive there because you were afraid of getting lost. You got to the city okay by train but then the taxi driver himself couldn't find the exam location and you were almost late and very anxious when you arrived, and very distressed when you eventually got home. I think you failed that element in the exam on this occasion, but you passed the retake.

This was about the time of the currant bun incident (I should explain to people in the United States that a currant bun is functionally something like a muffin). You knew I liked currant buns and bought some on the way home from work, but the bag slipped off the car seat and underneath the brake pedal, and rather than squash them you drove into the car in front, which was being rather slow in taking the double bend just before our house. Then you hit it again because it was still going rather slowly. When you brought the other driver to the house, he was a nervous wreck.

For seven years you worked as a psychiatrist, part-time because you knew you needed not to overtax yourself. You were also undertaking a further programme in psychotherapy. Another of your favourite movies was *Truly, Madly, Deeply*. You loved the movie because the therapist in it was so good at just sitting there listening, and holding back from speaking, while the bereaved Juliet Stephenson character simply talked. As years passed, you yourself talked less and less, until eventually you no longer spoke at all, but even by nature you were not a loud mouth like me, and when you did speak it was likely to be something worth weighing and pondering. Of course I never saw you in the therapy room, but I imagine you being able to hold back and encourage a person to talk, and then being able to speak things worth heeding.

Psychiatry is a profession suspicious of Christians (the suspicion is mutual), but you were fortunate that there was a tradition of Christian involvement in psychiatry in Nottingham and you had a number of Christian colleagues. But your supervisor, in particular, seemed suspicious of you, though I came to wonder whether that was because he sensed that mentally you weren't functioning as well as you needed to do in this demanding profession. You had to give a paper to the postgraduate seminar and had decided to give it on 'Values in Psychiatry', but you couldn't get your mind around the subject or around how to write a paper, so we wrote it together, and eventually published it under both our names.

You would come home each day needing to offload the troubles and worries of the situation, and would pour them out as we sat at the table after dinner when the boys had gone off to play or to watch TV. I think it was a tricky time in my own work, and I felt you weren't interested in me and my life and needs. So this was a time when the illness started taking its toll on me as well as on you. I had trouble sleeping (I think maybe you took sleeping pills) and I would get up in the middle of the night to sit on the sofa and cry out to God about it.

Physically, too, things got tougher. You were finding it harder to drive the car. We bought an automatic and a foot control to move the gas/brake pedal to your left foot, your better foot, but you never drove it. By some route that I cannot remember, you were required to take a physical examination by the British equivalent of the DMV and they determined that you could no longer drive.

Losing that freedom was one of the more painful stages of loss involved in the progress of the illness. You started going to the hospital by taxi, which worked okay.

A couple of years ago I asked Mark, who as our younger son had lived more of his childhood with his mother being ill, whether he thought it had affected him. In the back of my mind was an occasion from when he was about eight. You had been in hospital not because of the MS but because you had a lump in your breast, which turned out to be benign. Your mother was staying with us and she said something to Mark about 'When mommy gets better', by which she meant when you came out of hospital. Mark said, 'Mommy will never really get better.' For twenty-five years or so I lived with those words, wondering what it was like for him to grow up with that awareness. I think it may have been another visit to you during the same hospital stay when I also had a conversation with Steven (who would have been about eleven) that stayed with me. For some reason just he and I were going to see you, and as we drove along Derby Road I asked him whether your illness worried him. 'Well, yes, it does, rather,' he replied from the back seat of the car. The trouble was I didn't know where to go next with the conversation.

Adapting

When I finally had the courage and the opportunity to ask Mark about growing up with his mother being ill, the taxi featured. He seemed to know what he wanted to say in reply to my question; I think his wife Sarah had probably asked him the question. He didn't feel it had been a terrible burden; the way our life was, was simply the way our life was, even if it was different from other people's (which is also how it has seemed to me). Maybe it was no odder than being brought up by a psychiatrist and a minister. He went on to recall how we used to go swimming on Saturdays (which we started doing for your sake, because swimming was a good form of exercise for you), followed by fish sticks and fries in the leisure centre's cafeteria. He also recalled an occasion when he had slept late and missed the school bus; you made him come with you in your taxi, which you diverted to go via his school. Those were Mark's ways of saying that your illness didn't stop us doing family and that your mothering may have been different from other people's, but it was real.

From time to time you would fret over your mothering and would recall that nurse who declared that you had no right to have children. I would reply that living with your illness would be the making of Steven and Mark as it had been the making of me, and I think that has been true; at least, you have every reason to be proud of your two sons and no reason to think that they grew up bitter and twisted. Admittedly I have just hinted at another factor in what has made them the men they are. They both married great women who I think are the kind of people who get them to talk about and talk through whatever they need to talk about and talk through. Both sons married in the last year we were in England before moving to California; when you have got your sons into the hands of good women, I often say, you can flee the country.

We started using a wheelchair occasionally during the early 1980s. Students often ask me which has been my favourite rock concert, and I usually tell them about two from this period. I know little about the music of those years when we were bringing up children and juggling careers, but in about 1984 Steven and Mark had reached the age when we could take them with us, and we went to see both Dire Straights and Eric Clapton at the National Exhibition Centre near Birmingham. For the second of these, you sat in your wheelchair for the walk from the car with the intention that you would transfer to a seat when we got inside, but the security people took one look and said, 'I'm sorry, Madam, if you can't really walk, you can't sit in an ordinary seat', and conducted us down to the front where we sat about five yards away from the band, able to see the sweat on Eric's face if he ever broke out into a sweat.

In general, however, for me this was one of the toughest periods. I couldn't imagine how I could continue coping with the loneliness of carrying the burden of living with your illness and the aloneness. I don't mean that other people failed to support me, but in the end it was my wife who was sick. There was a Graham Kendrick song we sang in chapel a lot during this period.

> In your way and in your time,
> That's how it's going to be in my life.
> And in your perfect way I'll rest my weary mind
> And as you lead I'll follow close behind,
> And in your presence I will know your peace is mine.
> In your time there is rest, there is rest.
>
> In your way and in your time,
> That's how it's going to be in my life.
> Dear Jesus, soothe me now till all my strivings cease,
> Kiss me with the beauty of your peace,
> And I will wait and not be anxious at the time.
> In your time there is rest, there is rest.
>
> And though some prayers I've prayed
> May seem unanswered yet
> You never come too quickly or too late
> And I will wait and I will not regret the time.
> In your time there is rest, there is rest, there is rest.[1]

Invariably I sang the song in tears wanting to mean it, aspiring to mean it, knowing it was true, wanting to believe it.

Retirement

In due course one late winter afternoon at the beginning of 1988 your boss, Richard Turner, came to our home to see us, to say that he thought you needed to retire because of the state of your health. Your problems with memory and other mental functioning made it unsafe for you to continue working (for instance, with the authority to prescribe drugs). You accepted this more easily than I might have expected. You used to quote a line from the missionary and spiritual writer Amy Carmichael: 'In acceptance lieth peace.' With a nasty irony, in St John's Theological College I became principal (in US terms, a cross between being president, provost, and dean) on the same day that your retirement took effect, 1 April 1988.

Someone commented that maybe you would now have a ministry among our seminary students in counselling or in teaching counselling, but the effect of the illness made that unrealistic as it made continuing to work as a psychiatrist impossible. Instead, without trying, you began to have another kind of ministry. You had long accompanied me to the main evening chapel service each week; now I started taking you into lunch each day and you became more of a consistent part of the theological college's life. When your mother died, with some money from her estate we had a lift fitted on the main stairs so you could more easily reach the chapel and the dining room on the upper floor of the building.

You loved the students in St John's and you had an extraordinary capacity to arouse love in them. An incident sums it up for me. We went to our friend Scilla Yates's for dinner. At the end of the meal, you were enthusing over the cheesecake, and Scilla offered to put some in a doggy bag, and did. Then after dinner you asked her whether she had any chocolate to go with our coffee (a fine British custom). She didn't have any, but thought for a moment or two and then set off on foot to buy a (large) block from a gas station. You had behaved in the situation in a way that lacked inhibition, an almost childlike way, but one might think it was actually the proper human way, as you let Scilla behave in the proper human way, with an expression of a deep love and acceptance of you. It is normal to love knowing something that another person whom we care about really wants, because we can then get a kick out of fulfilling their want. But we hesitate to reveal the little things we really want, so we deprive the other person of the thrill of fulfilling this desire. So you blessed people (including me) in giving us the chance to do things for you.

Therefore I am sorry that I would sometimes get annoyed with you, particularly if you expressed your discomfort or tiredness as apparent annoyance with me. But I am aware how most of the time you were capable of smiling with as much happiness in your eyes as I ever remember. Even though you grieved over your loss of independence and your inability to work, you lived life moment by moment, often enjoying the surprises that come to someone who will not remember what was supposed to happen next.

In about 1993 you had a massive seizure caused by an infection. Only afterwards did I know that this was what had happened; I simply awoke at 3 a.m. one morning because you were violently convulsing. I called 999 (911 in US-speak) and within minutes a doctor had come and given you a shot that stopped the convulsing, but you spent a week in hospital lying in bed unable to control your movements or speak, simply waving your hand uncontrollably. Your neurologist assured me that you would get back to your 'normal', which I found hard to believe, but he was right. A few weeks later when we went for a follow-up appointment I told him that I had found his promise or prediction hard to believe, and he told me he had found it hard to believe too, but it was what the textbooks said should be the case, and they were right. From then on you had a urinary catheter, which mostly dealt with the problem that had led to the infection, though it made you liable to other minor infections. You began to take anti-seizure medicine and never had another major 'tonic-clonic seizure', though every few months you would have a little seizure that just involved your face distorting a bit, and it would usually stop after a few minutes.

We lived in a three-story principal's house with six bedrooms and our sons had by now both left home. Phil and Sue Groom were students who had studies in the house for a while and so saw more of you than most. Sue was later working for a doctoral degree looking at formation for ministry and she comments that knowing you in this period was a large part of her formation for ordained ministry. You taught her so much by the way you lived your life. You taught people to enjoy life and to stop and look and wait and watch and accept and be. Sue and Phil lived on a narrow boat on a canal and one of Sue's memories is of a time we took you for a ride on the boat, which involved putting cushions on the side of the boat so we could slide you from the quay onto the boat itself. My other memory of that afternoon is the way the boat travelled at about four miles per hour. This drove me mad. I could cope with standing still or moving at eighty miles per hour, but not with a canal boat's snail-like slowness. In contrast, you loved the way you could observe every blade of grass. I realized again how people who live more slowly can get more out of life.

I had long assumed that about ten years was as long as I should stay as principal, and as that decade passed I came to feel this on my own account as well as on the theological college's. The way I picture it is that I was carrying final responsibility under God for St John's during the day, but then when I came home in the evening there was no escape from responsibility. I had to decide everything there, too.

THE LAST YEARS OF YOUR MINISTRY

Over a decade or two, Fuller Seminary in Pasadena had asked me two or three times if I was interested in a post but we had never taken the inquiry seriously. The first time, we had talked about it with Alan Murphy as your physician, and he had advised against moving to the United States where the pace of life would put more pressure on you in your work. Yet there had seemed no reason to say 'Please stop asking me', and eventually Fuller was again looking for an Old Testament professor at the time I was coming toward the end of that ten year period. One bright September morning, the Dean of the School of Theology called to raise the possibility once more. While work pressure on you was no longer an issue, I barely knew where Pasadena was and specifically knew nothing about the Californian climate except that the sun shone; as far as I was concerned it was the same as Florida, hot and humid, and we knew that heat and humidity took it out of you. Fortunately the dean had a relative with MS and knew a little about the disease. 'But it's a desert climate,' he said. Suddenly something apparently impractical became a possibility. We knew that warmth combined with low humidity was good for you. It's always humid in England even when it's cold. We used to go on holiday in the summer in the French Alps, and one year you cried because you couldn't walk as well after we got home as you could in France.

Losing Speech

We came to Pasadena for an interview in April 1997 and immediately you could move more easily than you could in Nottingham. We found a lovely open-space ground floor apartment that would work well for us if I did accept a job here. Admittedly, you didn't want to leave Nottingham. You loved our house and its garden with its birds and squirrels, you appreciated your caregiver Janet Clarke who was so loving, and you enjoyed your friendships with the students, but I think the biggest factor was that you just don't like relocating. I reminded you that you hadn't wanted to leave London to move to Nottingham, and now you didn't want to leave Nottingham. There were other practical risks involved: I didn't really know how your medical care would turn out given the big difference in the two countries' systems. But I had to bet on the fact that God and circumstances otherwise pointed in the direction of making the move.

There was one snag about the apartment: it had a pile carpet that you were not going to be able to navigate. That became irrelevant when in June you had a relapse of the MS that finally terminated your capacity to walk. We celebrated Mark and Sarah's wedding on 16 August, had a family farewell celebration the next day, and on 20 August drove to London Airport to fly to Los Angeles. My vivid memory is of dropping you at Heathrow. When I was transferring you from the car to the wheelchair, you couldn't help me help you. The nurses had taught me to balance my knees against yours, but in trying to do that in swiveling you from the car, my knees lost contact with yours and you buckled to the floor. To my relief there was a shout from outside the terminal doors, and there were the rest of the family waiting to meet us and able to help get you up.

Settling in California was extraordinarily uneventful. By email we had already made contact with a couple of potential caregivers; in the first day or two we interviewed and appointed them. Over the next weeks you moved from 'I don't want to leave Nottingham' to 'It's not as bad in California as I expected' to 'I quite like it here' to 'I think I like it more than England.' We were soon having visits from family and friends, whose memories record how happy and settled you became. Anne Long commented on your smiling eyes that reflected the sun, and your sense of humour and fun (she remembers a time I danced you in your wheelchair and how you enjoyed that; I don't remember the occasion, but it seems entirely plausible), and she remembers the love that poured out of your eyes even when you couldn't speak. Fuller staff member Barbara Bell smiles to remember early dinners in our apartment with you engaged in dinner table conversation and laughing at me.

Two or three years after we moved, you lost the ability to swallow and over a period of months spoke less and less until you didn't speak at all. As results of the MS, both problems were neurological rather than physiological. It wasn't that you knew what you wanted to say but couldn't move your lips to say it. Your difficulty lay in working out what you wanted to say. I fretted about the implications this had for your relationship with God. Could you relate to God if you couldn't work out what to say? Words are so important to me. Some time later a student commented, 'I always wonder if people like Ann have a special communion with God in their silence. I hope so.' I hoped so, too, but I had no conviction about it. There was no evidence of it. I feared that maybe it was not so at all. More often I assume that silence was simply loss, and that this is the price you paid for ministering to people. There is no theological reason why it should be the case that God has a special communion with people in their silence. God is ruthless about using people for the sake of others even when it brings no benefit to the people themselves. But if so, I knew that God honoured your ministering thus, and I knew that when you and God decided that enough was enough, God would say, 'Welcome, good and faithful servant; come into the joy of your Lord.' I nevertheless expressed my worry to Cathy Schaller, who pointed out the fallacy in my assumptions. God could commune with you spirit to spirit even if you didn't have the words to use. Later, Francis Bridger also commented, 'I am amazed at the deep structures in our connection with God at the level of human-divine spirit, especially perhaps when the ill person can't speak.'

Speaking without Words

The United States is a postcolonial culture, which means it has a love-hate relationship with its European background. I am mostly the beneficiary of people's undue regard for a British accent, which makes them assume I am talking sense, and I am the beneficiary of students' appreciation for my quirkiness, lack of dress sense, and inclination to question ideas that they hold dearest and that they assume are biblical. Commenting on this in the words I quoted at the opening of this book, Erika Haub then added,

> 'What I did not expect was to have my life changed by the mostly silent woman who sat in a wheelchair who was his wife. Ann Goldingay was a steady presence in my Fuller experience. So much of what John was bore the mark of her life impressed upon his. As he would teach, it often felt as if she were there in the classroom with us.'

Another student commented

> 'I was thinking last night as you talked of Ann that even now she continues to minister to others. I know that if I were in her place I would want my life to affect others, to make them think and to stir their hearts. I am grateful for sharing her life and your life with her.'

In England we lived on the theological college campus and students were always in and out of our house. Because the arrangement in Fuller is very different, we had to think of different ways of being able to get to know students, and we fell into the habit of inviting them for tea and scones. The fascination with Europe played into this. You shared your scone recipe with your Indonesian caregiver, Yanti, who later shared it with her Kenyan successor Rahab, who shared it with her Filipino successor Chel, who shared it with her Chinese Filipino successor Christine (throughout our time in the United States we have had great caregivers); the scones became very multi-ethnic. Erika continues,

> *'I remember the first time I was in their home, sitting somewhat awkwardly by her side, speaking with her without expecting any verbal response. I remember John turning toward her with a smile and a funny comment when she would seem to cry out in the midst of a class visit.'*

The cry will probably have meant you were trying to cough and having difficulty in doing so. Erika goes on to recall a September night when her husband and I and another guy carried you in your wheelchair up the steep flight of stairs to reach their apartment in South Los Angeles to join in a surprise celebration for her birthday. Actually, I hauled you up and down stairs a lot, often on my own, and it gives me a bit of a chill to recall it, because I could easily have lost control and dropped you down the stairs; but it never happened.

Amy Meverden reminisces about the first time she met you when she came for a BBQ by the pool.

> *'Ann was sitting away from the table. I picked up one of the students' babies and brought her with me to sit in a chair near Ann. At first I was so occupied with the infant that I didn't notice Ann craning to get a good look at the baby. I*

lowered the baby to her level, and her eyes sparkled. I called another student to bring over the other infant who was at the BBQ, and Ann was clearly delighted. I was so moved by the love that I witnessed in her eyes. I wondered if these babies reminded her of her own sons, of her grandchildren, of the babies she oversaw during her years of medical residency. I wondered if their presence made her happy, or if it pained her to see infants of such a delightful age and not to have the ability to fold them into her arms. From that point on, Ann's presence had a lasting impact on my life. Her presence would trigger my imagination. I would wonder about the life she lived, about the pain of such a brilliant and innovative woman trapped within an unresponsive body. I felt guilty, that I, a single woman with no husband, no children and no career, had full physical capabilities, while a psychotherapist, wife and mother sat nearly motionless in my presence. I thought about you [Amy is referring to me], and the pain of having to witness the love of your life degenerate.'

Helping People Face Weakness and Fear

Your friend Sol Nuñez used sometimes to come and sit with you when I had to be at a meeting and one of the caregivers was not due to be with us. In a chapel talk she spoke of what she has learned through you. On this occasion, as you sat with her at the front of chapel, she shared an excerpt from her journal, written as if she, too, is speaking to you. She describes an occasion when she came to sit with you.

'You whimpered and cried for a while. John wasn't there to take over or make it better. We were alone, you and I. As I held your hand, I could not help but feel helpless.

Helplessness! I do not like that word; much less the feelings attached to it. My worldview teaches me to be in control, to be strong and independent. I can compete with the best of them and be successful. I don't need anybody. I work hard at what I do and I can pull myself up by my bootstraps. But, Ann, you are helpless, vulnerable and fragile. By your very presence, you bring out those fears in me. And I realize that my world really isn't that safe and I am not as much in control as I think I am or as I want to be. In that helplessness I began to sing, and holding hands with you, I realized we were not alone. I was with you and you were with me and God was with us. In your discomfort, in my song, in our clasped hands, we three were together. Then peace came over your face and to my heart. Emmanuel! You teach me that to be human is to live in a world that is neither perfect nor safe. You invite me to trust God and live my life in complete dependence on Him, in whom we live, move, and have our being.'

On another occasion Sol observed, 'Ann teaches me that to be human is to experience vulnerability, weakness and fragility. She invites me to embrace all of my humanity; the strong, stable parts along with the weak, fragile ones.'

Another student also comments on her fear.

'I visited the Goldingays' home quite often during my first year or two at Fuller. I often felt uncomfortable when I approached Ann to say hello because I didn't know what to say to someone who could not speak to me, but I wanted to push past my fear and acknowledge her just as I would any other person. At times I felt distant from the others who frequented the Goldingays, most likely because they were cultured, articulate, and intelligent. When they spoke about theology, art, films, and music, I really didn't have

> a lot to add to the conversation. When I finally did have something to say, I remained quiet and paralyzed. I had been silent for so long that it was hard to change the pattern. This was strange for me, because I consider myself an extrovert and fairly social. I realized that there was no longer just one Ann Goldingay in the room. I began to feel what it must be like to be Ann, with so many thoughts and feelings being experienced, yet at the same time an inability to communicate them. If there was anyone in the room that I could relate to, it was Ann. I wished someone had acknowledged me, the silent figure at the dinner table or around the TV in the midst of a bustling conversation. I wished that someone could have seen that my silence did not mean disinterest or stupidity. It was scary to identify myself with Ann's seemingly lifeless figure, but by doing so I experienced a silent solidarity with her. For that experience of being able to relate to Ann, I am grateful.'

Theologically, what this pushes people towards is a centredness in grace. Another Old Testament professor, Gerald Janzen, puts it this way as he remembers coming to lecture in Nottingham. One of the 'indelible memories' he took away, he said, was of you in your wheelchair 'so clearly held in everyone's affection, and yourself communicating a centredness in grace'. Communicating this centredness must say something about your inner being, something subjective within you. It also says something about who you are objectively. There is a sense in which you have no option but to rely on God's grace. You can't do anything. You embody the fact that it is possible to be a human being and not be able to do anything. It is not doing that constitutes you; it cannot be. You are constituted by grace. You remind people that God embraces us in our brokenness and our limitations, and you do this especially as you affirm a centredness in God's grace not a dependence on what you do. And further, you draw love from people. Stanley

Hauerwas has commented that we don't want to be faced by people with handicaps and chronic illnesses. If that is true as a generalization, then many people in our Christian communities (church and seminary) and in our secular communities (jazz clubs and restaurants), prove glorious exceptions. You draw love out of them, love for you and also for me.

Not Able to Tell Us

For the first third of its time, our marriage was quite ordinary (well, insofar as a minister/theologian and physician/psychiatrist could ever be ordinary). For the middle third, it was tough. There is a sense in which, oddly, it then became ordinary again. I came unconsciously to accept it as ordinary or normal for us. It is what it is, weird by other people's standards, but normal for us. While I do look after you, we do the things other people do (well, except that they don't). We go to two or three concerts each week. We have people to dinner and we go out to dinner. We go to the beach for lunch most weeks.

There are things we don't do. Only once since we came to the United States have we got on a plane. But that's fine; there are worse places to be stuck than Southern California. We no longer go to places where there is no elevator because I have become afraid that one day I will lose control as we haul you up or down stairs, or that I will put my back out. We have given up going to movies, partly because you can no longer lift your head and I'm not sure you are able to enjoy the movie at all, so we watch movies at home on DVD where your recliner chair makes it theoretically possible for you to see the TV screen (though I am not sure you are actually able to focus on it). Going out for music is a selfish indulgence on my part, as it helps keep me sane, but I can also rationalize that music reaches the parts other things don't reach; there is at least a chance that you are enjoying it. I do mostly take you to things where they play the kind of music you will enjoy—no heavy metal, and no freeform jazz because long ago you told me you like music that sounds as if it's going somewhere.

I could easily feel that a grey-haired man accompanying someone in a wheelchair is out of place in many of the clubs we go to. Yet people never make us feel unwelcome. I remember the time two hefty bouncers lifted you onto the wings of the stage at the Troubadour in Hollywood because they didn't think you would be able to see very well from the floor. I said this to someone and she commented that our life simply illustrates the nature of marriage: 'two people just hanging on to each other, for better for worse, because this is who we are and what we do'. She went on to say that as a stance it was 'countercultural—counter not only to the culture of the world, but of the church too'. We aren't trying to give some Christian witness to the nature of marriage. We are just being married. What else could we do? But if it comes across as countercultural in a positive way, I am grateful that you make me do it.

It's really hard not being able to know what you like and what you don't like, what you are thinking. I often say that we will spend the first ten years in heaven with you telling me all the things I did wrong. I appreciated it when someone said that on the contrary you will want to spend the first hundred years telling me all the things I did right. Hazel Michelson reminded me about something that happened when we came to Fuller for the interview and my now-colleague Leslie Allen invited us all to lunch at his house. You were in the wheelchair, unable to climb the steps. As you watched me go with Leslie to open the doors you turned to Hazel and said, 'He's a good man.' 'Yes, Ann, he is,' Hazel said. Do you carry on thinking that? There are reasons you should, and reasons you shouldn't.

More recently, Steve Mann sent me this message:

> 'As I was driving home tonight, I suddenly was hit with a
> strong feeling that I should pray for Ann. I've never felt so
> compelled to pray something. I remembered your chapel

message on God intervening, and I went with it. I prayed
for Ann's healing. Then I was in your house, and Ann was
in her chair, and I said to her, "Hello, Ann." But it wasn't
me speaking. It was a quiet, assured, perfectly toned voice. I
can remember it vividly, and I want to say that the best
description for that voice is love. I said it once more, "Hello,
Ann," and there was a smile in my voice. Just twice. I think
it was Jesus' voice. I've never heard anything so assured,
like everything is okay. Then I was overwhelmed for about
an hour (it is a good thing my drive is two hours) and I am
quite sure that I was feeling Ann's love for you. She is so
proud of you, and so in love with you. So there I am, driving
with tears streaming down my face with Ann's love for you
coming out of me. I saw myself writing this email telling
you this picture. I think it is an answer to prayer. There.
That's it. I've never had anything like this happen to me
before. I'm only a Quaker.'

Teetering on the Edge

The next to last time you caught pneumonia was in 2008. For some
weeks you had seemed to be in some discomfort and agitation,
and then the pneumonia was diagnosed. You had two forms of
antibiotic and they were having no great effect. On a Thursday
the doctor said she was willing to try another, though she didn't
think there was any point; she left me to think about it. I found
myself saying to God, 'I know Ann has a ministry, precisely in her
weakness. But how long should it go on? I don't have it in me any
longer to prolong it. I shall not ask for yet more antibiotics. If you
want her still to exercise her ministry, you will either have to give
me a sign, or do it yourself.'

Later that day I had good conversations with Steven and Mark,
who were both happy with the stance I was taking, and Steven

told me how he had just been reading C.S. Lewis's *Chronicles of Narnia* with his son. There the boy resists the witch's suggestion that he should give the apple to his mother who is sick rather than giving it to the lion as the lion had said. The lion confirms that the apple would have brought healing to the boy's mother, but says it would not have brought her happiness in the long run. On the Friday, your nurse said that the trouble with more antibiotics was that it might do damage in the long run. I wasn't asking for divine confirmation that my stance was right, only for divine disconfirmation, but I got the thing I wasn't asking for.

All this encouraged me in my conclusion that if you and God wanted you to recover, it was between the two of you. Humanly-speaking the chances were small, and Steven and Mark started thinking about air tickets. On the Saturday you started to improve. On the Sunday I took you off the regular oxygen machine for us to go to church and took the portable oxygen container with us, but you were breathing okay and I never put you back on it. A day or two later, the doctor pronounced you quite well, but I hardly needed that affirmation. You were brighter and more alert than you had been for weeks. I was quite shell-shocked, in a good way. Francis Bridger later commented that 'the capacity of those who are seriously ill and unable to speak' (even facing death) to determine that 'now is not the time' (along with God) is remarkable.

God had acted to keep your ministry going, and you had agreed to take it on again—or the other way around. Amy Drennan testified to it a few weeks later after a chapel service in which we had celebrated Holy Communion. You couldn't receive the actual bread and wine, of course, but I asked Amy to come and pray for you.

> *'When I touched Ann to pray for her and offer her the body*
> *of Christ, she jolted. I really felt she knew me, and was*
> *responding to this offering of Christ that we were extending.*
> *It was a deeply relational moment for me. I felt she gave*
> *me a small gift, an offering of life to our body of Christ,*

and a reminder to me that God embraces me through my
limited and broken self. I thought of it later in the context
of Todd Johnson's sermon about recognizing signs of life
in the midst of tragedy, sickness, and the like. I felt deeply
sorrowful, I remembered your sorrow, yet I knew God's
presence with us in blessing Ann, and God's reaching out
to me through Ann.'

Some months later, after a baccalaureate service (the farewell
service for graduating students), Matt Lumpkin sent me a message:

'I was videoing the service, as I usually do, and listening as
Linda Wagoner was recalling aloud the beautiful symmetry
between the Genesis and Revelation readings about living
water springing up and trees for food and for healing and
how we groan in longing for new creation. You were seated
behind Ann in my shot and I noticed that you were rubbing
your eyes. I began to wonder if you were feeling particularly
moved by these passages (as I was) or if you were simply
experiencing allergies (as I also often do). A few seconds
later, I heard a deep, longing, desperate groan rise up from
Ann and fill the vaulted chamber, echoing through the
congregation. I was completely overwhelmed and undone
by the profound poetry and beauty of this moment. I don't
know if Ann intended to bear witness to her own longing
in this way or not. But either Ann or God or both of them
had something to teach me about this dynamic of life in the
tent of mortality. I hope you will thank her on my behalf
and accept my thanks for the way you both bear witness
to the hard struggle of love. Mine and my wife's marriage
is better for it. Thank you.'

I do remember rubbing my eyes, which I think was just allergies,
and I did hear your groan, and I assumed you were simply

trying to cough or something, but nevertheless it was indeed an expression of your incapacity and helplessness. Our daughter-in-law Sue remembers an occasion some years previously when we were pushing you in the wheelchair through Pasadena and you cried out, 'This is horrible.' My colleague Mark Labberton has commented that 'my experience as a pastor does not lead me to romanticize such circumstances' as the ones you and I have lived with, and an ongoing experience of disability like yours.

— 3 —

A Death and a Life

Ann died later in the month of that baccalaureate service, on the last Sunday in June 2009. (I now give up writing in the form of address to her).

Half of me had known the moment would come, yet Ann had recovered from pneumonia four or five times and I was quite prepared for her to keep doing this Houdini act for another decade or two, and maybe to see *me* off. So while one half of me knew this moment would come, the other half suspected it would never come. But come it did.

On Friday, once again she had a fever, but this sometimes happened and it didn't worry me too much, so we went to the Hollywood Bowl for Aretha Franklin as planned. The next day she was moaning a bit, which worried me more, but some Tylenol again did the trick and that evening we went to the Los Angeles Arboretum for George Gershwin as planned (and if I spend the last two nights of my life at open-air concerts like that, you won't hear me complaining; and incidentally, she was wearing an Eric Clapton tee-shirt when she died, which would also be okay for me).

Early Sunday I could tell she was having a hard time breathing, and I took her to Urgent Care at about 7.30 a.m. They wanted to get her admitted to the Huntington Hospital, as they usually do, and I gave my usual reply that I had promised her and me that she wasn't going into hospital ever again and please would they get her stabilized and send us home with antibiotics and oxygen, like before. This always bemused them a bit, though they don't have much option but to agree, I guess, and they got in touch with the hospice agency to arrange for her to be admitted and thus for the agency to arrange for the oxygen. During the morning I was half-aware that she wasn't stabilizing so much. About 12.30 I was in the midst of leaving to be at home to receive the oxygen so they could send her home. There were two nurses and a doctor in the room, and suddenly one of them said, 'She's stopped breathing' and another nurse maybe looked across at the monitor where the lines were going flat like in a TV movie, and that nurse said, 'She's gone.' It reminded me of the scriptural phrase about giving up the spirit, giving the breath back to the God who gave it. Ann had breathed her last. For a moment or two the doctor and the nurses felt for pulses and things like that, but they knew we weren't due to go in for aggressive measures at resuscitation, and after a moment I asked them to leave me alone with Ann for a bit, and I held her, and prayed for her, and gave her to God.

Then it became a bit farce-like as they didn't really want this dead body around too long please, so which mortuary would come and collect it? Because we had been near this moment before, I had once worked that out, so I came home to get the information and call the mortuary, and call our sons, and call Christine who had been Ann's caregiver with me for the previous two years. She and her husband came to Urgent Care to be with me with Ann until the mortuary person came at 4 p.m. We sat with Ann and held her hand and prayed and felt her getting colder. It was very significant to have that long period of time with her as the shock came home. The man then wrapped her in a clean white linen shroud, again like the Gospel story, and we said goodbye to her body. I asked for her to be cremated so that I could take her ashes with me to England, as I had always envisaged I would, so that we could have a memorial service in the church near London where one of our sons belongs, and so that I could scatter her ashes in that valley where we had spent the first night of our honeymoon forty-two years previously and where I remember the happiness with which we went for that walk on the first morning of our married life, her in her little white dress with blue and yellow flowers.

'My Grace is Enough'

I was due to preach the following Sunday, but I asked to be excused, though if I had preached, the New Testament lesson from 2 Corinthians 12 that was set for that day would have been impossible to resist. In Eugene Peterson's paraphrase, Paul says:

> I was given the gift of a handicap to keep me in constant touch with my limitations ... At first I didn't think of it as a gift, and I begged God to remove it. Three times I did that, and then he told me, 'My grace is enough; it's all you need. My strength comes into its own in your weaknesses.'

Through her life she had served God and served other people, though in changing ways. For the first third of the years that she lived with MS, she combined with aplomb being girl-friend and wife and mother, student and doctor and psychiatrist, not to say clergy wife and professor's wife. Then the course of the illness had changed and she had gradually lost her physical capacities and her capacity for remembering things, so that for most people in California she was a silent figure in a wheelchair. Three times and more we and other people begged God to remove this handicap, but God said, 'My strength comes into its own in her weakness.' And things people had said and said after her death testified to the way she ministered silently to hundreds of people. At least two people flew from the other side of the country to be at her service in Pasadena because of what she meant to them, even though they never heard her speak. Another couple who insisted that she took part in their marriage service by sitting alongside me as I married them seriously looked into whether they could come from Beirut for the memorial.

For much of this time she was more content than in the years when she was relatively fit; she became less driven, less liable to anxiety. Nevertheless it had troubled me the previous year or two that she had sometimes seemed not quite so content and at peace as before, and I had thought, 'Lord, do you think she has fulfilled this vocation for long enough? Couldn't you let her rest now?' I didn't quite say this to God, because when I say such things, God is inclined to reply, 'What I do with Ann is between Ann and me, so shut up.' Perhaps God heard me anyway. But in her life, God's strength sure came into its own in her weakness. A day or two later, one of our friends in an email spoke of his 'vivid memory of the day you told me of Ann's illness all those years ago, and of your faith then that God was in it and with you and always would be'. Forty-three years previously that had been, and God had been in it, and with her, and with me, all the way through.

There was a hymn that I originally planned to have at the funeral and then forgot about, a hymn we had at our wedding, because it was a particular favourite of Ann's, by Kate B Wilkinson. It's a prayer that was pretty much answered.

> May the mind of Christ, my Saviour,
> Live in me from day to day,
> By His love and power controlling
> All I do and say.
>
> May the Word of God dwell richly
> In my heart from hour to hour,
> So that all may see I triumph
> Only through His power.

May the peace of God my Father
Rule my life in everything,
That I may be calm to comfort
Sick and sorrowing.

May the love of Jesus fill me
As the waters fill the sea;
Him exalting, self abasing,
This is victory.

May I run the race before me,
Strong and brave to face the foe,
Looking only unto Jesus
As I onward go.

May His beauty rest upon me,
As I seek the lost to win,
And may they forget the channel,
Seeing only Him.

When Was the Last Time?

A few months previously we had watched the movie *And When Did You Last See Your Father?,* a memoir by the poet Blake Morrison about his relationship with his father, and in particular about his father's illness and decline at the end of his life. It made me write a parallel poem, as if someone had asked me, 'And When Did You Last See Ann?'

Was it the last time she was able to raise her eyebrow?
Was it the last time she smiled?
Was it the last time she swallowed?
Was it the last time she laughed?
Was it the last time she said 'John'?

Was it the last time she cried?
Was it the last time she transferred to a pew in church?
Was it the last time she signed her name?
Was it the last time she could complain at what you were doing?
Was it the last time she could give herself something to eat?
Was it the last time she decided what she would like for dinner?
Was it the last time she could walk?
Was it the last time she could remember her address?
Was it the last time she said 'No'?
Was it the last time she slept in the same bed as you?
Was it the last time she could climb stairs?
Was it the last time she could go to the bathroom on her own?
Was it the last time she took part in a conversation?
Was it the last time she decided what to wear?
Was it the last time she could get you a birthday card?
Was it the last time she used the phone?
Was it the last time she prayed out loud?
Was it the last time she made love with you?
Was it the last time she read a book?
Was it the last time she argued with you?
Was it the last time she drove the car?
Was it the last time she used the computer?
Was it the last time she gave her testimony?
Was it the last time she went to work?
Was it the last time she cooked dinner?
Was it the last time she took a photograph?
Was it the last time she could wash and dry her own hair?
Was it the last time she danced with you?
Was it the last time she could cut your hair?
Was it the last time she played tennis with you?
Was it the last time she wrote a paper?

With all those, I never knew it would be the last time until afterwards, when she never did that again. I had wondered, what other 'last time' could there yet be? What is there left? I was now in a position to answer that question. When Did You Last See Ann? It was the last time she breathed.

You never know it will be the last time until afterwards, when she never does that thing again. There are two or three couples of about our age whom I sometimes see walking about near where we lived, holding hands or just being together. One is a couple I know, and I stopped them one day and said, 'Don't take for granted that you can walk around like that.' There is another couple whom I sometimes watched dancing at one of the clubs we would go to, and one evening I said to them, 'Don't take for granted that you can do that.' One time it will be the last time. I guess there is a touch of envy about my response to them, though only a touch. Mostly it's something more like wonder. It resembles the feeling I have when I watch our sons and their wives doing marriage, relating to each other as people who love each other and are each other's friends and work together and accept each other in a relaxed way with their foibles, and on one hand relating to their children and on the other to their niece and nephew. It reminds me of the way Ann and I once were, when these two young men were themselves children, and while it's capable of drawing out some sadness, more dominant is a sense of wonderment and joy.

People's Memories

From time to time over the years I have received emails from people commenting on what Ann meant to them, and when she died, I received a load more, as well as messages in letters and on greetings cards. It's hard for people who knew her only in her latter years to imagine her as a person full of regular human strength, full of drive and energy, as she was. Among the words that were used to describe her to me during the days after her death were feisty, insightful, determined, caring, funny, gentle, courageous, warm, thoughtful, sparkling, and deep. Graham and Molly Dow commented, 'We thought of her as humble: although well-qualified in medicine and psychiatry she never gave the impression of having superior knowledge.' Morag Fowler described her as 'a bright spark'. Elaine Labourel called her 'quite a lady' and added, 'I remember when you came to dinner—it must be twenty years ago—and Ann told me I ought to be a Reader; and I'm a Rector today. There's discernment/prophecy for you.' Another description was 'incredibly polite', which just shows you how a married couple can have complementary strengths. (And I know she sat up on the morning of her Memorial Service in Pasadena and said 'John! You can't go to my Memorial Service in shorts and a pink shirt,' and I said, 'Well, you took off, dear, so you surrendered the position to influence what happens.' But in the end I put on my long pants.)

Erika Haub commented on the passing of two giants since she had left Fuller Seminary, New Testament professor David Scholer and Systematic Theology and Pastoral Theology professor Ray Anderson, 'two giants of faithful instruction at Fuller and beyond'. Soon afterward she could have added Geoffrey Bromiley, world-famous Systematic Theology professor before Erika's time, who died just after Ann. Erika goes on,

> 'Ann too was a giant, and her life instructed so many of us. ... As I have thought about Ann these past days, I have been struck by a passage in Philippians chapter one that for me describes the kind of impact Ann has had on my life. The apostle Paul writes of a different sort of bondage than that which robbed Ann of her movement and speech, but the truth of how that bondage impacted others is the same. He writes:
>
> '"I want you to know, brothers, that what has happened to me has really served to advance the gospel ... Because of my chains, most of the brothers in the Lord have been encouraged to speak the word of God more courageously

and fearlessly ... Yes, and I will continue to rejoice, for I know that through your prayers and the help given by the Spirit of Jesus Christ, what has happened to me will turn out for my deliverance. I eagerly expect and hope that I will in no way be ashamed, but will have sufficient courage so that now as always Christ will be exalted in my body, whether by life or by death. For to me, to live is Christ and to die is gain. If I am to go on living in the body, this will mean fruitful labour for me. Yet what shall I choose? I do not know! I am torn between the two: I desire to depart and be with Christ, which is better by far; but it is more necessary for you that I remain in the body. Convinced of this, I know that I will remain, and I will continue with all of you for your progress and joy in the faith, so that through my being with you again your joy in Christ Jesus will overflow on account of me."

'... I can testify with certainty that there are significant riverbeds of progress and joy that wind through my soul as a result of Ann Goldingay.'

Charles Read commented on the funeral service of a mutual friend at which my former boss Colin Buchanan had preached on the line from Hebrews, 'Though dead, yet he speaks.' Charles commented that this is true for Ann too, and that 'indeed in these latter years it has been true that "though silent, yet she speaks".'

The Two of Us

Almost from the beginning at Fuller I took Ann to chapel. We had sat in the back row on the right where we could put the wheelchair at the end of a row. Then over the last four or five years I took her into the seminary much more, to meetings, events and lunches— in fact to everything apart from classes (except maybe once or twice when I had a sudden caregiver emergency); if she were in class, I didn't think I would be able to concentrate for wondering if she was okay. I think I started taking her to other things because of the ill-health of one of our caregivers (who in fact died before Ann), but I thought that anyway being with me in meetings was likely to be no more boring than sitting at home, and maybe more enjoyable because she was with me. Then I realized that being around the seminary more made it possible for her to exercise her mysterious ministry to people. People I didn't know would stop us on the way across the campus and say hello to her. To me, there was nothing extraordinary about taking her with me, as I did to the beach and to jazz clubs, but for other people it was unusual; there was no one else wandering about the campus, pushed in a wheelchair. I took for granted the unusual nature of our relationship, but it was less instinctive for other people to do so.

Many of the messages I received after Ann died concerned their response to the two of us, arising in part out of our being present in the seminary in this way. My problem in this section of the book is that the messages are therefore about me as well as Ann, and it is somewhat indecorous for me to share them. I can only ask the reader to bracket that fact and work with the further fact that anything people say about 'us' or about 'me' is true only because of 'her'; anything about me is about the effect she had on me. Doug McConnell, dean of one of our schools, commented to me that 'each time we have talked about your ministry in our Fuller community, you credited her.' That's true, and I was not being falsely modest. Virtually anything that I am, in some sense I am because of Ann. Hazel Michelson said: 'Long after your students have forgotten what you said, they will remember what you were'—because of her. Mark Labberton, who arrived as a professor at Fuller at about the time Ann died and never met her, moved into what had been my office (with some irony, Fuller had got me to move to a different office that was wheelchair-accessible; Ann visited it twice). He commented, 'It doesn't take long to hear stories, and even more to see the evidence in people's eyes, that your love for one another was a very special gift. I sense the significance of all this for many at Fuller.' Our friend Sue Groom observed, 'One of my fondest memories of Ann is of when we came to visit you in Pasadena and Ann sat in her chair with little apparent reaction to anything until you came into the room and her face lit up and she beamed at you. That spoke so much to me about the power of love.' Dottie and Fred Davison said: 'You and Ann gave meaning to the word marriage.' Colin Moody emailed: 'Every Wednesday, both of you were there in chapel worshipping together, living out a love beyond words. Seeing your life together deepened my appreciation for human love and for God's love.' A student told me just before he graduated that he and his wife were having a very hard time adjusting to married life but that watching us and knowing about us helped them persevere. Jeremy Trew commented, with British humour:

> 'Thirteen years ago, Alison and I were about to get married. We needed a special licence to get married in the St John's chapel, and you had to sign on the form that you would take us through appropriate marriage preparation. Our conversation went something along the following lines: You: "It's so long since I did this, I'm not sure what I'm supposed to do." Me: "Me neither, we don't cover marriage preparation until next term." You: "Well, when you've done it tell me what I'm supposed to do and we'll do it." I don't recall any formal marriage preparation ever happening, and like most newly-weds we had our share of arguments as we learned to live with each other, and maybe more importantly, we learned that we couldn't live without each other. John, your marriage preparation sucks, but the relationship you and Ann shared, and shared with us, was plenty good enough. You two lived out something well beyond romantic love, though that was there too. That was

> *the love which carried one another's burdens and tries not to count the cost; a love that hopes; a love that remains when the waves retreat. That was good theology—grace and more grace.'*

A student whose father had been abusive to her family and unfaithful to her mother, which eventually issued in their divorce, wrote:

> *'I believe that God placed you in my life to help me heal. Though you write in* Walk On *about struggling with infidelity, you repented and saw the error of your ways and mourned your actions. You moved on and committed to love Ann in spite of past indiscretions. You ended your life loving Ann more than any other human could have conceivably loved her. You made mistakes, but you displayed for me an example of a husband laying down his life for his wife. This was something that I had not directly encountered before witnessing your marriage. More than your contribution to biblical scholarship, your presence as a skilled lecturer, your ability to deliver moving chapel sermons, your eccentric wardrobe color schemes, your day-old-breadcrust-dry humor, your advanced barbequeing/scone-making skills, all the encouragement you showered upon me in my studies, the lies you told in the letters of recommendation you wrote on my behalf, or the friendship you so willingly offered me, your gift to me was the ability to witness your day-to-day decision to love your wife, even in the most painful of circumstances.'*

I have to apologize again for the way this section may seem to glorify me. Of course I am moved by people saying things like that, but I have to say again that the point about including it is to help the reader see another significance in Ann's life, in what she drew from me.

What I Learned about the Old Testament through Ann

Soon after Ann died, Lisa Lee Miller in Singapore urged me in an email not to stop talking about Ann in class. I said I didn't realize I talked about her much. Lisa fell about laughing (insofar as you can do so in an email). I realized (I think) that she was referring in part to my speaking of things I have learned through Ann and ways in which the Old Testament has impacted my life through her. Students ask me why I came to be involved with the Old Testament, and I can give various true and/or funny answers to that (like that it was the first subject in the degree programme; if Church History had come first, I would have been a church historian). But then I tell them that the question why am I still passionate about the Old Testament is a different one. The answer is that the Old Testament speaks so powerfully about real life and about living real life with God; and our shared dealing with Ann's illness is a large factor in causing it to do so for me. So this is another way she has impacted people and will continue to do so, because there is no reason why I should stop talking in those terms. Before she died, another student commented, 'as you shared your life, and your life with her' in speaking that way in class and 'blending' life and scripture, 'even now she continues to minister to others.'

When people ask me what is my favourite book in the Bible, I say Ecclesiastes (this is not the right answer; you are supposed to say John or Romans). I wrote some years ago about Ecclesiastes (in the Guidelines Bible Reading Notes published by BRF):

> My wife Ann is lying on the sofa at the other end of the room, to safeguard against getting pressure sores. A few weeks ago we received a Christmas card from one of her psychotherapy patients (now herself a therapist), who remembers the sessions she had with Ann and looks back on them as a decisive shaping influence on her life. Today Ann cannot remember what

country she lives in, nor what day it is, nor what are the names of the two caregivers who have shared in looking after her for over two years, nor what is the name of the grandson who brought her such joy when he was here a few weeks ago. She is unable to swallow or to speak. She was watching the television news, though I am not sure how much she takes in. On that news we had been hearing of the terrible cost of the Russian invasion of Chechnya, of the suffering of the local people and of the Russian bodies surrounding their tanks. The pictures were too grim to show us.

In a moment I will take her out for a walk in her wheelchair in the warm winter sun, and we will have an ice cream, and if we are lucky she will be able to eat a little of it, and as I push her back up the hill to our apartment I will sing silly songs and pretend I am not going to make it to the top, and she will laugh. It is not enough, but it is not nothing, and it is certainly not to be despised. It is a gift from God. That is what Ecclesiastes says.

Just before Ann died, Matt Lumpkin wrote

> *'A classmate of mine and I have both heard our wives remark that we are better husbands during the quarters we are in your classes. I don't know exactly all that they mean by that but I suspect it is in no small part due to the reminder you offer to cherish the little joys, the brief and fleeting wondrous moments that still spring up in the midst of stress and difficulty. Indeed, the "problem" of blessing is greater than the problem of evil.'*

In that last remark he is referring to a comment I sometimes make when people are fretting about the problem of evil. It's odd that people who are not suffering often seem to fret more about this problem than people who are suffering. And it's odd that they are people who each day have food to eat and sunshine to enjoy and friends to share life with and a roof over their head and God to talk to. What on earth are we to make of the fact that there is so much good in the world? Isn't that at least as striking as the fact that there is so much suffering and evil?

Being Human

I recognized that Lisa was right. It is also the case that I often refer to Ann in unplanned ways because I realize that she provides an illustration of a particular point. But here are two further examples of things I always make a point of saying.

First, in lecturing on Genesis, I discuss what Ann's being made in God's image tells us about God's image. Genesis suggests that humanity was made in God's image in order to share in governing the world on God's behalf, and disabled people share in that; so they draw our attention to the way poverty, vulnerability, and weakness can have a mysterious power to move and transform, and they remind us how activity occupied God only for six days, not for seven; we are Godlike by inactivity as well as by activity. They remind us that life is a journey, a becoming as well as a being, and though that may not apply in the same sense to God, we can see in Scripture how God operates in different ways in different contexts; God's 'I am who I am' or 'I will be what I will be' points to this fact. God's having a unique name (which is revealed in that connection) reminds us of God's unique individuality, as our individual human names reflect the unique individuality of each human being—which includes the disabled. From 'in God's image' Genesis goes on to 'male and female', which reminds us that we are designed to live in relationship; and disabled people remind us of that fact in being more often driven to live in relationship, being more obviously in no position to live in isolation. Then, an image is intrinsically physical. Made in God's image, we embody what God would be like if God were a physical person; and disabled people have to deal with being physical and are less free to evade it than the rest of us.

Second, on her blog concerning Ann, Erika Haub included this quotation from something I wrote (in *The Usual Suspects /Walk On*) on Job:

> What we may be able to infer is that calamities do have explanations, even if we do not know what they are, for there is another feature of the story of Job that delights me every time I think about it, not least because it establishes a similarity between Job and us. It is that Job himself never knows about chapters 1 and 2 of 'his' book. So he goes through his pain the same way we do. And he illustrates how the fact that we do not know what might explain our suffering, what purpose God might have in it, does not constitute the slightest suggestion that the suffering has no explanation ... I cannot imagine the story that makes it okay for God to have made Ann go through what she has been through. But I can imagine that there is such a story.

Someone responded to Erika's blog by speaking in particular of things of mine they had read. I'm not sure precisely what paper their comment refers to, but that doesn't matter so much. The point is, it was evidently something I had written which they knew I couldn't have written if it had not been for Ann.

> *'Although we have not known the Goldingays personally, we understood even from our distance that Dr Goldingay's ability to speak into our circumstances was a direct function of his experience with his wife. We are forever grateful that she paid the price of her discipleship because she stands tall in a very small group of fellow-believers who have worked for our comfort and edification, instead of for harm. Her direct contribution to our ministry is one of the greatest*

gifts we have ever received. All of life changed after our discovery of one paper in particular—it had been night and suddenly it was day.'

At Ann's memorial service Tom Smail commented that Ann stands in different ways behind all that I write, including the abstruse academic things. I have mentioned that I helped Ann write a paper about values in psychotherapy when she could no longer articulate things very clearly. The way she helped me write vastly, vastly exceeded that. She stands within the frame of everything I write, sometimes visibly, sometimes invisibly. She drives me back all the time to basic questions about what it means to be human with God. When it is some other context that presses a question, she provides key elements in the subconscious framework within which I think about it. In important ways I failed her but at least here I acknowledge her.

— 4 —

WITHOUT HER

A little while after Ann died, a colleague whose wife had died a year or two previously gave me the name of the therapist who had helped him process his grief, and I thought I might call her at some stage, but I never did so, mostly because I prefer spending my spare time and money on rock and roll. Instead I started journalling what was happening; that helps me process what is going on. I became aware that the experience of bereavement and grieving was a changing one. Every week, then every two weeks, then every month was different.

Week 1   (28 June – 4 July)

An agitated two weeks. In the end, Ann's death had been sudden. Perhaps the time that immediately followed would have been agitated even if that had not been so, but certainly with its being sudden it was a shock, even though it had been threatened for years. So I guess I was a bit traumatized and needing to assimilate and start coming to terms with what had happened, while at the same time having to do things that needed to be done. I was somewhat manic about doing these things, and that was an expression of the agitation and the associated internal turmoil and energy.

The morning after Ann died, Christine and I sorted out Ann's things. I had read that you aren't supposed to throw away all the belongings of the person you have lost, which was just as well as I am the thrower-away in the family and I would probably have done so. Initially I planned simply to keep the nice clothes, but in the end I kept everything. We did throw away anything that related to Ann's illness, or sorted them to take them to the convalescent care charity. There were pills, catheters, diapers, rubber ring, IV stand, formula, patient lift, folding commode, and so on, and so on. In addition I phoned the agencies to which the hospital bed and the wheelchair belonged, and brought Ann's own bed up from the downstairs storage room in our complex. I put her bed where mine had been and moved mine to where hers had been. That was partly convenience, as her bed was nearer the door and the bathroom, but maybe it was partly associating myself with her. Apparently some people wear their loved one's clothes after they die, which seems a bit weird; this was perhaps my equivalent. (I had planned to sleep in Ann's bed, but I had forgotten that it too was a special one, with rubber covering, which would have been very hot, especially in June. I wondered how this had affected her.)

The Sunday Ann died, we were going to Laguna Beach for lunch, so after Christine and I had sorted things out on that first Monday, I went to Laguna on my own for lunch and then drove back for my class in the seminary in the evening. This all now seems really weird, but it seemed logical at the time. I had emailed scores of people with the news about Ann on Sunday evening, and when I came back from Laguna there were about eleven phone messages from people who wanted to sympathize or drop by or bring me food (or were actually at the main door of our complex carrying the food). I had various other offers of food over the next few days, some of which I failed to evade; I eventually discovered that it is US custom to bring food to someone who has been bereaved. I was relieved I had missed the people who left the messages or dropped by. I knew I needed to be on my own to begin that process of assimilating what had happened, and people use up so much energy.

On Tuesday morning the agencies showed up for the bed and wheelchair, and in the afternoon I took the other things to the convalescent aid charity. I also wanted to dispose of our van, which was adapted to take the wheelchair. I fancied something like a Honda Element or Toyota Scion; in the 1970s and 1980s we had three Renault 4s and these look a bit like the Renault 4. I wonder if I was trying to get behind the illness to the happy years when we had those; I have a number of photos of Ann with each of them. But at the Honda dealer I happened to spot the Honda Fit, which as a hatchback was a bit like our UK Ford Escort. It also thus had happy associations, and it was cheaper to buy and run.

By late Tuesday nearly all traces of Ann's illness had gone. Maybe this was too fast. For some weeks afterwards it gave me a shock to open the cupboard where the meds had been and find it empty except for things such as coffee that I started keeping there. After some time I noticed that we still have the little corner cupboard near Ann's bed in which we kept some things that we used every day in connection with her needs (I wrote 'we' still have it; I wonder how long it will take me to stop using the first-person plural). I left it there; maybe I will think of some things to put in it. But trashing all the things that were related to the illness felt and still feels a good kind of repudiation of the illness that had so circumscribed Ann's life for such a long time (as I type that, I cry). You are supposed to be angry when you lose someone; that was as near as I got to anger.

On the other hand, someone suggested maybe it was a blessing that she died, and in my email message I had said I was glad for her that she can sleep until resurrection day and awake renewed. I am not sure who this person thought Ann's death was a blessing for. I had wondered myself whether I would feel relieved that at last it was all over, but I have not felt that at all. Oddly, ten years ago, or fifteen, or twenty, maybe even twenty-five years ago, I would have been relieved. I would not have been able to face the idea that this would go on for all these years. But over the most recent years I have become more and more accepting of the nature of our life together and have come to assume that Ann would quite likely live as long as me, and I have looked forward to that prospect (in fact, my concern has been how I would cope with looking after her as I got frailer). That's related to the way over the last four or five years I had been taking Ann into Fuller more, so that in effect we had presented as a couple. I had liked that fact, not least because I knew she exercised her ministry by that means. I had grown to love her more just the way she was, even while feeling grieved and guilty that I could not put it right, and guilty about whether there were ways I might hurt her as I heaved her around, or bore her by places I took her to.

Whereas on Sunday I had emailed the seminary to say I thought I would probably take the week off, on the Monday morning I felt I would rather teach my class and maybe have time off later. In some ways that was a sensible decision; over the following weeks it was good to have something normal to do and I appreciated having the structured meetings with the students each Monday and Wednesday evening. In the classes I often alluded to what was going on and how I felt about things, which felt helpful to me, and is the kind of thing students love (I only half-understand why that is so). On another level no doubt I needed to draw breath. While I felt I was okay to teach on the Monday, I knew I had an infection. I was muzzy and had a slightly sore throat. It was presumably the infection that Ann had had, and on the Wednesday it knocked me flat for the day, so that I had to withdraw from the class. No doubt that was partly my psyche saying 'Excuse me, I need to stop for a moment.'

I arranged with the seminary to send a note around the faculty about Ann and to put a note on the internal website, and arranged with our rector, Antony Miller, to have a memorial service the following Monday. On the first occasion when it had seemed likely that Ann would die, I had imagined having a memorial service in the seminary; indeed, I had made tentative arrangements along these lines with relevant people. But somehow that no longer seemed appropriate; I don't really know why, though the fact that it was summer vacation was a part of it. I told the faculty about the memorial service but didn't put out a public notice, partly because I didn't want to imply that people should come, partly because I was afraid too many people would come for our little church. So I just told people who asked. As a consequence, some people who didn't ask and thought there would be a public announcement missed the service and were a little aggrieved.

On the Thursday I felt physically much better and drafted a eulogy for Ann, whose contents appear one way or another in this book. I came across the poem 'When Did You Last See Ann?' which I had written a few months previously, and wondered whether to include it, being unsure whether it was more about me than Ann. I incorporated it in the draft I sent to Antony as we planned the service and asked his advice, and he urged me to leave it in.

That day I also went to the dealership where we bought the adapted van, and the man who had sold it to us apologetically offered me half what I had paid a couple of years previously, which was nevertheless almost the list price of the new Honda. I went to a blues concert in a park for half an hour or so in the evening. I didn't want to have people visiting me, nor did I want to speak to them on the phone, but after I had spent time on my own at home, I appreciated being in human company in the evening for a little while without having to relate to anyone. On the Friday I emailed the director of the Pasadena Jazz Institute, where we often listened to jazz, to tell him about Ann and to say I would be there for an hour that evening. Showing up at things without Ann when people weren't expecting this seemed hard; I preferred people to know ahead of time. I don't mind people then talking to me about it and expressing sympathy; I just preferred them to know before I arrived. I did the same later with other places we used to visit often.

Saturday was Independence Day. I went back to Honda, test drove the Fit, proved I could remember how to do a gear shift, and signed to buy it.

Week 2   (5–11 July)

During much of these first two weeks I felt okay, though numb and empty. I didn't eat much, though I did eat some brownies and cherry pie filling, leftovers from our Hollywood Bowl picnic the Friday before Ann died. Once or twice a day something would bring the horror home and I would break into a howl. One example was the Fuller Human Resources people calling (in response to a message from me) to talk me through making necessary adjustments online to my insurance cover. That involved me in pressing the delete button in respect of Ann. I had to delete Ann.

On the Sunday I robed for church but told Antony I would probably rather not preside at Communion, though when it came to it I felt okay about doing so. The space in the back corner of the church where Ann would sit in her wheelchair was empty because she was not filling it, and it stayed empty for weeks. There was no reason a chair should not be put in the space; perhaps church people unconsciously left it because it was Ann's space. That first Sunday its emptiness screamed at me and I thought it might do so for ages, maybe forever, though after a few weeks it stopped doing so even though I was still aware of it, and after a while church people started putting a chair there.

In the evening that first Sunday I dropped by a friend's birthday party at another concert in the park (I had been due to organize the party, but had been relieved of doing so) to stay just for an hour. On the Monday we had the memorial service at St Barnabas, which was a great occasion. There were enough people to pack the church but not to need an overflow. I robed. I don't remember what Antony said in the sermon. Christine contributed nicely and bravely after my eulogy, as did the former rector's wife, who knew Ann when we first joined St Barnabas and she could speak. The women of the church organized a fried chicken lunch.

The mortuary still hadn't got from the physician the signature on the death certificate that would make the cremation possible, but I agreed with my son Steven that we needed to go firm on having the memorial service in England on the Friday and that if necessary we would proceed without the ashes. I wondered about waiting to fly until Thursday night or Friday morning to allow an extra day (and I could teach my Wednesday class), but Steven wisely said this was risky; it would be odd if the plane got delayed and I was not there in time. So I booked a ticket online for Wednesday, with some complication over paying for it (I can't remember the details) so that I had to talk to a nice woman in Auckland and pay an extra $100. Then the undertaker called to say they had the signature and the cremation could proceed (another $50 for speedy action on that front). We collected the ashes on the way to the airport and I arranged for the Wednesday class to see a video of a lecture given in a previous year (which I had also done on the day I was sick).

It was great seeing our sons Steven and Mark and their families, and the people who came to the service and the reception. There were people who had been with me in the youth fellowship fifty years ago, people from Ann's medical school, former St John's faculty, and former St John's students, as well as family such as my sister and her husband and their son, and some cousins. Steven and Mark read the lessons from Psalm 73 and Philippians 2. These were tough passages and they found them tough; I admired them for reading them.

Next day we drove up to Dovedale and had lunch at the Isaak Walton Hotel, where Ann and I had spent the first night of our honeymoon. After lunch we walked up the valley by the side of the stream. I found the walk very hard because it took me back to our doing that walk the first morning of our marriage, with such happiness. We went just past the stepping stones that many people were using to cross the stream, as Ann and I had done that first morning, to a meadow where there were fewer people, and I scattered the ashes into the river—they mostly came out altogether so it was more like throwing them. Steven and Mark joined in and Steven took photos. Afterwards we climbed the hill on the other side of the valley, Thorpe Cloud, the hill Ann and I had looked out at from our bedroom early on that first morning.

The weather was overcast but warm (if it had been sunny, it would have been too hot). We walked back to the hotel where we lounged on the grass and ate the exotic pastries that we had bought on the way. They are called Elephant's Feet, because they seem almost that size and have something of that appearance; they are made of choux pastry, cream and chocolate. Before we moved to California, on a Saturday morning I would say to Ann, 'I'll take you anywhere in the world for lunch,' and she would say, 'But I want to go to Bird's Café in Wollaton,' a mile or so from where we lived, and we would go there for a baked potato and chili followed by one of these pastries, shared between us. They are at the top of the list of things about England that I miss.

Weeks 3 to 4   (12–25 July)

As I came back to Los Angeles from London, I was aware that now the real thing starts. The first two weeks had been full of necessary activity. That was now over and the real coming to terms could begin. I was on my own for that. I realized that bereavement is like getting married. For two weeks there is lots of activity and attention from other people. Then the time when it is all over as far as they are concerned and they go back to getting on with their own lives is the time when for you the real thing begins.

A colleague later commented that it was very odd to see me without Ann. I have noted that over the previous four or five years we had been more and more inseparable. For pretty much everything except classes, we were together—in the seminary, at church and in leisure. We thus unintentionally presented as a couple, an odd couple who embodied what it means to be frail and helpless and what it means to be married to someone like that. So what does it now mean to be me on my own? One aspect of the question concerns my own sense of identity, a question I had long recognized would arise if Ann died. Looking after her had been the centre around which my life focussed; so now my life has lost its focus. The newer aspect that I recognize in light of the way things have been over recent years concerns the way we presented publicly. We had a joint ministry, and it may have been more significant than my ministry as scholar or teacher or pastor. Making sure Ann could exercise her ministry had been a very significant part of what I had been about. So what is the nature of my ministry now? How do I present now?

This question was highlighted by people's messages after Ann's death. They expressed their sympathy in varying ways. As well as bringing food, they phoned (which I didn't care for, because I never liked the phone much), or sent cards, or emailed (which were both okay). Their cards and messages expressed standard traditional words of encouragement (theological or religious and otherwise), reminding me (for instance) that Ann was with Jesus; I didn't object to those, but neither did they encourage me. Some comments included a different kind of message of encouragement expressing insights that have also become standard, words that noted how I must be feeling loss, anger and puzzlement. These I found annoying; they felt like one-size-fits-all pieces of pop psychology and as a matter of fact were not always accurate descriptions of what I was feeling. The messages I appreciated were ones that expressed something concrete about what Ann had meant to the person who wrote. Some were brief, some longer; a number appear in this book. Every one of these messages made me cry, in a good way, yet in a way that vastly heightened my sense of loss and bewilderment about the future.

The day after I came home, Steven commented in an email that he had been overwhelmed by things people had said to him about Ann, or had written in emails, or had written on cards. They had made him see her from a different perspective, because to him she was 'just my mom'. I was thrilled that to him she was 'just my mom', but I was also thrilled that he had got to see her from this other perspective. To my surprise, over the next few days I too became overwhelmed by those messages about the way Ann had affected people. A number were from people in the seminary whom I do not know or hardly know, or people who had not even met Ann but who learned of her story. I had often thought and said that her having her ministry to people helped to take the edge off the awfulness of the illness, but in the back of my mind I had also wondered whether I was exaggerating its significance to make me feel better. Now it transpires that I didn't know the half of it.

That realization makes even more pressing the question of what I am to be about from now on, if my key vocation has been letting Ann exercise her ministry and that vocation is now over. Although I did not feel angry at her death on my own account (or my anger is repressed, if the pop psychology is right), I began to feel something like anger at her ministry being terminated, as well as bewilderment about what the future means for me. At the same time I also think, and I have to remind myself that I had been thinking, that her ministry was becoming very wearing on her and I had been asking how long she had to continue fulfilling it, and that I am glad for her to be able to rest until resurrection day.

One interim view of my future vocation that I reached was that I simply 'retire' in the sense of 'withdraw' into my academic work, into writing and teaching. There is quite enough there. It is a form of retirement in the sense that my significant lifework is over. Another was that I needed to be prepared simply to face the future and discover what ministry God had for me. It was a question of living open to possibilities. The past is the past; who knows what the future might be. A friend who lost her husband some years ago commented,

> *'It may take you time to adjust to the great empty space that has opened up for you. Your life has been emptied in one way, but will now, if gradually, be filled with new life as you enter a new chapter of your life. This great space can be intimidating at first, particularly in your case. Give yourself space and time to move into it gently.'*

Weeks 5 to 6   (26 July – 8 August)

Weeks 3 to 4 had also been the weeks I couldn't sleep. I would drop off okay, but wake up after an hour or so and not really settle again. I didn't get hopelessly overtired because I would sleep on the patio in the afternoons, but it was wearing. I was also conscious that my brain wasn't functioning very well. I wasn't thinking very quickly. In class I was having more trouble than usual formulating sentences and turning my outline notes into oral paragraphs. I also struggled with being able to write. A neighbour pointed out that the doctor could easily enough prescribe some sleeping pills, but that seemed somehow inappropriate. My insomnia was part of a proper reaction to Ann's death, of a recognizing of its reality, of recognizing her importance and my loss. In Old Testament Israel and in other cultures people fast and go about looking dishevelled (smearing their faces with dirt and tearing their clothes), and these are ways of ritualizing and formalizing a lack of interest in food or in one's appearance, a lack of interest in life; not being able to sleep is a parallel phenomenon. At the beginning of week five I googled 'insomnia' and as a result more or less gave up coffee, tea and wine, and my sleep returned, though maybe that was partly coincidence; I later resumed caffeine and wine okay. I also resumed being able to write.

I received a phone call that week from a Fuller graduate working as a chaplain in Iraq who had been part of the Bible Study group at our house. Two Sundays previously he had felt compelled to preach on the idea of God's steadfast love or covenant love. He remembered my explaining one evening the Hebrew word that represents it, the word *hesed*, and my saying that I thought the best English word to convey the biblical idea of *hesed* was the word *commitment*. He added that as I talked about this I was at the same time feeding Ann her formula down her feeding tube, and what struck him was that we weren't just talking about love or commitment; it was something that was being acted out. (I am again embarrassed that this is a story about me, though I think of it more as a story about Ann and about something God did through her illness, and I ask you to think about it that way.) He told this story in his sermon. A few days later one of the soldiers who heard the sermon was killed in a mortar attack, and the chaplain had to pray with him as he died. He was so glad that the last sermon the soldier had heard concerned God's commitment and loving kindness.

The following Sunday the set psalm was Psalm 51 and in my sermon in connection with the psalm's opening appeal to God's 'steadfast love' I told this story. A woman came to talk to me in tears afterwards because since childhood she had been given a deep conviction that God was so full of wrath. She couldn't internalize the idea that God was characterized by grace, commitment and compassion. As it happened, we were studying David in class the next night, so I told the story again.

In the midst of this sequence of events, Lisa Lee Miller wrote to comment on what Ann had meant to her and her husband Gunnar.

'She graced our lives and taught us much more about grace,
love and life through her presence than most textbooks

full of words that teach about such things! I hope you will share Ann with future Fuller students who have not had the privilege of meeting her. Please keep telling aspects of her story in your classes. I loved hearing them, even the ones where you had more questions than answers about what God was up to in her life.'

Suddenly I saw connections between all this. Ann's dying did not mean I would stop talking about her. I have mentioned earlier that I was surprised when Lisa said I used to talk about Ann so much, but I can imagine she is right that I did, and I can imagine that I shall continue to do so, not least because of things I came to perceive theologically through her. That is part of the answer to the question how I shall present in the future, and part of a response to my sadness at my not being able to continue facilitating her ministry. I can still do so. Yes, though being dead she can still speak.

In general I thought I was now on a fairly smooth upward trajectory of recovery from the bereavement. (I wondered what is an appropriate word to describe this process, and I don't like the medical model suggested by 'recovery'. Yet the sense of brokenness and the painful emptiness are like the symptoms of an illness.) One or two people had commented in the past that I had done a lot of grieving for Ann when she was alive, and thus when she died I might not have as much grieving to do. Our hospice social worker had said I would probably find I didn't need to keep Ann's stuff as long as other people did. I felt slightly proud of my trajectory: I am a guy who copes. I don't mess around. I get on with things. I move quickly. While in some ways I am very un-American, in other ways I am quite American; I get on with things, I get things done. In our culture people often expect you to get over things, to get on with your life. If people ask how you are and you answer, 'I am doing okay,' that is the right answer. Generally, the question does not invite the response 'Well to be honest I'm just overwhelmed by the sense of being empty and of everything being pointless.'

I thought maybe I was indeed moving on and thus coping with the experience in a way that matched who I am. Yet I also felt a bit guilty. Shouldn't I be sadder for longer about losing Ann?

Weeks 7 to 8   (9–22 August)

At the beginning of the seventh week I suddenly felt down and depressed, and I was like that for Monday, Tuesday, and Wednesday. On Thursday I awoke with the third line of a song (written by Danny Whitten and recorded by Rita Coolidge and Rod Stewart) running through my head:

> I can tell by your eyes that you've probably been crying forever,
> And the stars in the sky don't mean nothing to you, they're a mirror.
> *I don't wanna talk about it, how you broke my heart. ...*
> ... I don't wanna talk about it, how you broke my heart. ...

Ann broke my heart twice. She did it as she gradually became incapacitated through her illness. She has now done it again by dying. I have noted that I didn't feel angry at her dying, and I still don't feel angry, but I am heart-broken. The man in the song doesn't feel angry but he does feel heart-broken. I don't understand why the other person has also probably been crying forever (is there a dialogue in the song or is this also him?), but for me it speaks of Ann's loss too.

Maybe I didn't want to talk about this or think about it. I just wanted to get over it and move on. Reflecting on it now, I realize that I had not previously thought of Ann's death in terms of having my heart broken. I'm not sure I had thought in those terms in the past in connection with her illness, though I used to say that it was as if she had left me. Since her death I have thought in terms of shock and loss and emptiness and pointlessness and aloneness, but having your heart broken is different. I don't mean I feel resentful towards Ann. Although objectively speaking she broke my heart, she did not do so deliberately. Now I see that her death broke my heart and that her dying is the end term of the heart-breaking process that had been going on for more than twenty-five years, and although I feel quite glad for her, I feel sad for me. When I realized the dynamics of the process whereby subconsciously I needed to own all this and that my being down was a sign of it but that I 'didn't want to talk about it', I laughed and wondered whether facing it would mean my spirit lifted; as it did.

I have been reading Romans, and I came to Paul's comment that 'Whatever was written ahead of time was written to teach us, so that through endurance and through the encouragement of the Scriptures we might have hope' (Romans 15:4). The Scriptures often portray the people of God having to put up with experiences they might wish did not come their way, but they put up with them—Jesus is the climactic illustration of that. All this contributes to the achievement of God's purpose to bring about the world's salvation, so that the Scriptures thus inspire us to endurance and hope. Perhaps I have to stay with the heart-brokenness rather than leaving it behind, in order to be able to minister in a way that encourages people? Oh, thanks. A student commented after a class when I had given my lecture on the image of God and handicap, 'One of the reasons the lecture works is that it issues from your reflecting on actual experience.'

I received a phone call from someone asking if they could speak to Ann. Such phone calls are always from people who don't personally know her—for instance, people at the doctor's office. When Ann was alive but unable to speak, it was always slightly problematic to know how to reply to them, and the calls were always a little painful. Now they are more so. On the other hand, I would still sometimes forget that Ann was gone. After I had been working at my desk for some time I could suddenly think 'Is Ann okay? I haven't spoken to her lately.' I would look up, and her chair is empty. I would also feel a little more horrified at how her death happened. Should I have spotted earlier that she was sick? Did I really have them burn up her body and did I really throw her ashes into a river? (I also reflected on the fact that cremation only hastens a process of destruction that in any case happens when we bury someone.)

Weeks 9 to 10 (23 August – 5 September)

Related to those questions is what difference it would make if I had had her buried and if I was in a position to visit her grave. I know some people go to the grave to talk to the person they have lost. Would I have done that? One Sunday about now, Antony referred to the possibility that the loved ones we have lost could be with us in spirit if not in body. It reminded me that Paul also refers to the possibility of being with someone in spirit when you are not with them in body. So I can project myself into the room where Ann is sleeping (her 'room' among the ones Jesus promises in John 14) and be with her. It involves my imagination, but it does not mean I am imagining something that is not real. I tried doing that and found it lifted my spirits. It is an act of true denial—that is, it denies that we are totally separated. In a way it works with the fact that our relationship over recent years has had quite a thin basis. It has involved me projecting myself into her life and her not being able to respond. So what is so different?!

I was aware that the Friday at the end of August would be two calendar months since Ann died, and it would be our forty-second wedding anniversary. It still seemed a bit unbelievable that she had died; but she had. Again I wondered whether the end of two months and the end of forty-two years and the way my trajectory had been maintaining a level path for two more weeks meant that the immediate aftermath of her death was over.

Then two days before that anniversary I awoke with a stiff neck. A couple of decades ago that used to happen from time to time, but I don't think it had happened since we came to California, and

I have been grateful to God for being protected from the kind of neck ache and backache that would have complicated caring for Ann. It was funny it should come now.

On Thursday I awoke at 6 a.m., still with a bit of a stiff neck and also feeling sad that no one will send me an anniversary card the next day. I would never have dreamed of sending an anniversary card to someone after their spouse had died. I would think it sensitive *not* to send a card. Yet I think I will always be aware that August 28 is our anniversary, and I would be comforted by someone else realizing this and realizing the particular sadness of the day.

On Friday I again awoke at 6 a.m., still with a bit of a stiff neck, and that morning our son Mark phoned, precisely because it was our anniversary. I didn't dream that either he or Steven (who was on holiday abroad) would do so. I was overcome by appreciation. I was able to tell him about the oddity I just noted about the way one feels on the anniversary.

When for the first time I went on my own to one of the jazz venues we visited most often, *Café 322* in the nearby city of Sierra Madre, I felt oddly distanced from the music. I found myself thinking, 'This is good, but what am I doing here?' I realized I was grieving, because it is a place where we had always gone together and it reminded me of her absence. I went there again for swing dancing on the evening of our anniversary and sat with a woman we often used to sit by, who like me says she can't do swing dancing but does rock'n'roll dancing. I could almost imagine asking her to dance.

One of the people who flew across the country for Ann's memorial, Amy, calls me or sends me postcards once or twice a week to check out that I am doing okay. This week, out of the blue, she told me I should not be dating for six months, and asked if I had been on *eHarmony* or whether in due course I would be. (There are circumstances in which I might advise a man who received from a woman such comments and questions to be a bit worried and careful, but for a variety of reasons I feel free not to be worried in Amy's case. To start with, I am older than her mother.) Through the years when it seemed likely that Ann would die when I was of more obviously marriageable age, I assumed I would marry again, and even in very recent years I could fantasize about it, but I now find it difficult to imagine. When Ann and I married, it involved a mutual commitment to form a new joint life, and one reason this wasn't so difficult was that as twenty-somethings neither of us had really formed our individual selves or lives. Then, the way things have been for over twenty years has meant that by default I have controlled the marriage. I'm not clear I am prepared to pay the cost of submitting myself to the kind of reshaping that would be involved in doing so again at this stage in my life. It would be delightful to have a friend and a lover, but I doubt if I am willing to pay the price, but we will see, after six months, or a year.

Not long before Ann died, we got to know a woman in her fifties whose husband had died a few years ago and who would say that she still felt married and couldn't imagine getting involved with another man. It would feel like unfaithfulness to her husband. She still felt committed to him. A mutual friend told us that the Russian Orthodox understanding of the marriage vows is that they are an adaptation of monastic vows: in other words, when people marry, they are saying to each other what otherwise they have said to God. Both for that woman and for me, for different reasons, he commented, 'the wedding vows have become monastic once again.' We were both living celibate lives not because that is our instinct or because it is natural to us or because we are made that way, but because that is our response to someone else (her dead husband, my handicapped wife). Our celibate lives were the giving of ourselves to this other person because of who they are, and also the giving of ourselves to people in general who become aware of it, see love expressed in it, and are thus blessed.

Weeks 11 to 12   (6–19 September)

I didn't write anything for a while and again wondered if the immediate aftermath might be over. I had decided a few weeks previously to have three or four days away in September; I thought it might be good for me. I then discovered that the other associate minister at our church was also feeling the need to have three or four days away, and we agreed to drive up Pacific Coast Highway to Monterey and back (about 350 miles each way). We set off on a Saturday and saw much amazing scenery. I slept a lot and I did lots of walking on beaches and climbing rocks, and ate lots of ice cream. Yet I was puzzled that most mornings I awoke feeling a bit down, wishing it was time to go home, and deciding that I didn't really like holidays.

I arrived home Wednesday evening and I awoke the next morning feeling definitely depressed. In a sense being away had taken my mind off Ann's having gone (though that recurrent feeling of being down indicates that my subconscious mind was still aware of it). I remembered occasions in the distant past when I would feel depressed after returning from a family holiday because the same challenges and issues that I had to face before the holiday would confront me when I got back. Consciously realizing this bit of dynamic again helped.

That day was the faculty retreat and I also realized as I arrived that this was going to be tough because I would be meeting many colleagues whom I had not seen since Ann's death, and many did ask how I was, or say nice things about Ann, or referred to the way they had been praying for me. The day started with a devotional reading from Luke 7:36–50 that involved our imaginatively entering into the scenes, and I never got beyond the passage's first line: 'One of the Pharisees asked Jesus to eat with him, and he went into the Pharisee's house.' As an evangelical and a theologian, I am a Pharisee. I am therefore free to ask Jesus to come into my (empty) house, and he will. After the imaginative reading, we were asked to draw our reaction to the passage or write a poem about it. I started a poem but realized that a visual image was the telling aspect to my reaction. Jesus was standing at the door of my house wanting to come in. I drew the huge doors of our complex and pictured Jesus standing there (I'm not sure why it was the outer doors rather than the door of our own unit). Then I recalled Holman Hunt's painting *The Light of the World* whose original sits in the chapel of my Oxford college, which takes up Revelation 3:20 with its image of Jesus standing at the door of our lives, so I drew that alongside the other picture, and opened my door for Jesus to come into my new life.

Week 13 (20–28 September)

A therapist friend had wondered what new things I might do now my life is so different. I was a bit nonplussed and didn't know what to say in response to this more positive and hopeful way of looking at the future than I could yet work with. Then one evening this week at *Café 322* I did dance, for the first time for more than twelve years (that is, since we came to the United States). It so happens that on one of the last occasions we went there before Ann died, the lead guitarist's girlfriend had asked if I would like to dance. She couldn't dance with her boyfriend because he was otherwise occupied and she could tell my body wanted to dance as I tapped my feet while sitting with Ann. I was touched then, but explained that because I couldn't dance with Ann, it would make me sad. It would also feel like an act of disloyalty. Now I danced.

Another stimulus to the drive to Monterey was to experiment with doing something new. Ann and I virtually never left the Los Angeles area and virtually never slept away from home because it was too complicated and because I would be anxious about something going wrong (Ann being ill, or the van breaking down, or...). I had more or less confined myself for some years to doing things she could join in. Although we can see mountains from our front door and there are many trails where people go walking in the foothills, only once or twice have I been walking there (on the first occasion, it was when two of our friends asked me what they could make it possible for me to do that I couldn't do because of Ann; and that was my answer).

While I could have placed her in a nursing home for a day or two so I could be away, I felt she would find that hard. More than one person has commented that when I enter the room, her face would light up, and the friend who sat by her in church used to say that she would suddenly pay more attention when I was leading the prayers or preaching. So I have felt I would be abandoning her by going away for a couple of days. I have thought about whether maybe I was exaggerating my own importance, and maybe I was, but that seemed a better risk than making her feel disoriented because I wasn't there.

Now that constraint is gone. I can go where I like. As well as driving to Monterey, I arranged to go to Princeton in October for a task force (which had previously met in Pasadena to make it possible for me to take part), to New Orleans in November (for an annual academic conference that I usually could not attend), and to London for Christmas (to stay with my sons). I have also been asked to go to teach or speak in Beirut, Toronto, Melbourne and Minneapolis, and have declined. I have realized afresh how much I actually appreciated her keeping me in Los Angeles. There are worse places to be confined, and I didn't have to think about declining invitations. Now, how shall I decide what to do? Initially I didn't want to go anywhere, but I think this instinct is subsiding, and although I agreed without enthusiasm to go to Princeton and New Orleans, in the end I enjoyed going (well, that's an understatement about New Orleans; I did find myself thinking I wished she was with me on Bourbon Street even though it's not exactly wheelchair-friendly). Years ago, I was an enthusiastic traveller. Maybe that sense will return, though this doesn't help with the decision about what invitations to respond to.

There have been one or two other new things that I have done. I had been to a soccer game at the Rose Bowl, the stadium within walking distance of our house; my grandson's team, Chelsea, were playing Internazionale Milano. I went to my first football game. In both cases I think one is enough; when you have seen one, you have seen them all (it would be different if it was my own soccer team, Birmingham City). I took different people out to concerts and clubs. When Ann died, I had tickets for us to go to eight summer concerts, so I took various people to these concerts in her place. Someone had a spare ticket for the upcoming U2 concert at the Rose Bowl, so I snagged that. I had never dared take Ann to the Rose Bowl; I was apprehensive about how it would work for her and for the wheelchair (though I had taken her to Dodger Stadium for the Rolling Stones and for Dave Matthews). Now I could go. I have been to other new music venues, particularly places that were upstairs and impractical for the wheelchair. I liked going to places where people did not have to wonder where Ann was and where I did not have to explain.

I arranged to have our kitchen mildly remodelled. The old countertops and floor were impossible to keep clean and the cupboards were showing their age, but I had postponed the work because it would be too much disruption while Ann was alive. Now I had the work done. I replaced the pictures that previously hung there with the paintings of 'The Four Seasons' by Pieter Breughel. We had bought these not long after we married and they had had a prominent place in three or four houses where we had lived. When we were packing things to come to the United States I thought we had lived with them for long enough and we would leave them behind, but one of our friends asked Ann what she thought about this and she was clear that she wanted to take them, so that settled it, and here they had hung either in our bedroom or in the guest bedroom for a further twelve years. Now they look down on me in the kitchen and remind me of what they meant to her. In general, I realized I liked being in our house: the kitchen, the sofa where I sit watching a DVD before going to bed, the recliner where I read the Bible and pray and journal, the desk where I write (but not so much the patio, where I sat so often with Ann; I cannot sit there yet).

I got into talking about bereavement with a student who had recently lost her father. She thought that the bereaved divide into people who can only think about the past and people who can only think about the future. She comes in the latter category and does battles with her mother, who comes in the former category. This is certainly where I belong; hence my appreciation when people write with reminiscences about Ann and my bemusement when asked what new things I might like to do. Yet I have found new things creeping up on me, and I can see that people who want to think only about the future need to think about the past; and people who want to think only about the past need to think about the future.

I do want to recapture the past that is lost. It is said that when someone loses their spouse after an illness, initially they can remember only the last months and this clouds over the happier times, but that eventually they regain their memory of the latter. I had thought that I might never do that recapturing because the times when Ann was well are decades ago. But some people's reminiscing about Ann relates to that time; they speak about her energy and her sense of humour. That has helped me; and I found myself wanting to have some photos on display from that time (for my benefit more than for other people's), and I have put up six by my desk. I have wanted to reinforce that memory. I was going to include one of her in a wheelchair, but in the end I didn't.

Related to this, one Sunday I ironed a tablecloth. It is just an ordinary tablecloth, but one we bought together and would use on special occasions; I think it was the only one that fitted our dining table, when it had its extension inserted for bigger dinner parties. We hadn't used it for years because it got horribly creased in the laundry. I don't think I had ironed since we came to California (who irons nowadays?—well, I don't). So I got it out of the drawer and spent half an hour ironing out the creases, then folded it and put it back in the drawer.

Month 4   (29 September – 28 October)

The day we reached the three-month anniversary of Ann's death, I again awoke feeling down; but I was also confident that it will be okay. Later, when I opened the file called 'After Ann' in which I had been journaling, it made Microsoft Word crash. When I re-opened it, the computer warned me that last time I opened 'After Ann', it caused a serious error and it asked whether I really wanted to open it again. I said I did. I had to keep thinking through the issues even where they were hard. Then in my day-by-day reading through Matthew I came to the story of a person who was totally disabled and was carried to Jesus (Matthew 9:1–8). Jesus said, 'Your sins are forgiven.' At first that made me angry. It isn't what Ann needs to have said to her. (Is it? Did her illness result from her sin? I don't want to think about that. Should I?) Then I thought about our action on that very day three months previously and pictured it as passing Ann on to Jesus, in the way this man's friends had done for him. We had been entrusting her to him. That very day Jesus had received her and said, 'Come, you who are blessed by my Father; take your inheritance, the kingdom prepared for you since the creation of the world' (Matthew 25:34; to collapse the difference between death and resurrection day for a moment). He would not have been able to receive her if he had not been prepared to say, 'Your sins are forgiven'; and he was prepared to say this among other things such as 'Come, you who are blessed.' In Ann's case (as in that of the disabled man in Matthew's story) this need not mean she is disabled because of her sin. It means that three months previously he welcomed her and accepted her as a sinner like the rest of us, and could therefore go on to say, 'Come with me and rest a while' until that day when he will say 'Get up and come home.' Once again therefore my sadness was mollified by an awareness that she is at rest and accepted. My concern with my being okay had been displaced by an awareness of her being okay; a joy in that fact means I am okay. In other words, for a moment I had forgotten my mantra 'sad for us, but good for her as she can sleep till resurrection day'.

For much of this month, once again I thought that I was doing so well most of the time that it was really all over; I was happy and positive and forward-looking. A weekend in the middle of the month exposed that I was wrong again.

One Thursday at *Café 322* I sat where we always used to sit; I had not sat there since Ann died. The following Saturday, hot weather returned after a day's rain and I decided to revert to my usual summer routine of sitting with my feet dangling in our complex's pool, reading a book, doing a lap of the pool a few times when I got too hot. I had not done that since Ann died because it was something I had never done without her sitting near me in the wheelchair. I enjoyed it, though I also felt a bit sad—but that seemed explicable. On Sunday I took Ann's shoes to church in connection with a project to collect shoes for people who need them; I thought I could handle starting to give away her things. At coffee after church, there too I sat where we used to sit; I had not done that since she died. Meanwhile, on the Saturday morning I had to give a 'meditation' at the 'Advisory Group' of the seminary's School of Psychology, and I talked about Ann, adapting my eulogy (material that appears in chapter 2 above). At the end, the Dean hugged me in thanking me, and I sobbed, but that seemed reasonable given what I had been talking about. On the Saturday evening I had a slight collision in the car (really only a fender bender), and this upset me more than it usually would.

But the weekend as a whole was dominated by the wedding of two people in our Bible Study group. It involved a rehearsal on Friday evening followed by a dinner, and by the wedding on Sunday followed by a reception. A number of people at the reception talked with me about Ann, and I wept a few times. Eventually I didn't want to be there any longer and halfway through, I excused myself and came home. Next morning I awoke still feeling down, though also knowing it was okay. I realized that subconsciously in the couple I could see Ann and me forty-two years ago. I think the man is a little bit like me in personality and the woman reminds me of Ann in her freshness and her joy in her love for her husband (and she is training to be a therapist). Looking at them as I took the wedding was like watching a video of our own wedding. At first I thought that what upset me was simply the wedding, but more likely it was the collocation over the weekend of events with emotional freight. Whichever is right, it showed that it was not over and I realized that probably this will not be the last time grief catches me out.

Something wild happened after a committee meeting. One of my colleagues asked me how Ann was. I replayed the question a couple of times in my head to make sure I had heard aright, then wondered whether it was a kind of metaphor ('How are you in relation to Ann?'). Eventually I said I wasn't sure what he meant. It transpired that he had been on sabbatical in the summer, had been ignoring emails, and didn't know about Ann's death. Ironically, about ten years ago when Ann had had her first pneumonia in May, it was he who had told me I needed to accept the fact that this was a sign of the end; she would certainly be gone by September.

Month 5   (29 October – 28 November)

At the beginning of the month I was asked to give a presentation via video streaming to the seminary's regional advisory board in Phoenix, and I did something like the meditation just described, but to match their request I made it longer by adding excerpts from the material that now appears in this chapter. When I finished, there was a strange silence. I realized that the chairman was weeping and unable to say anything; there was little verbal reaction from other people in the room, and he later told me they were weeping, too. One of them asked me if I was going to write a book along the lines of C.S. Lewis's *A Grief Observed*, which even for my pretentiousness seemed pretentious. I didn't think I had a book to write about it, though I did think there was an article, but if you are reading this, I was wrong.

Once again I thought it was nearly over. I no longer looked across our room and wondered why Ann's chair was empty. I no longer panicked that I hadn't spoken to her for the previous hour or so. Yet I came to realize that there was something new. I was fine as long as people didn't talk to me about Ann or ask how I was. I mentioned this to my sister, who told me that after my father died, my mother would cross the street to avoid meeting someone who would ask how she was. That expresses it perfectly.

Meeting with the task force at Princeton meant meeting with people who had known Ann from meetings in Pasadena and who naturally wanted to commiserate with me. I began to get messages from former students in England who had just had the news from the seminary newsletter, messages expressing sadness and appreciation for what Ann had meant to them. Our Dean of Chapel asked me to take part in our Thanksgiving service by giving thanks for Ann, and oddly, that somehow felt tougher than delivering the eulogy. Such experiences bring everything to my awareness again. In other words, it's there below, to be brought to the surface.

It's different with friends, when it's part of an ongoing relationship and they inquire how things are going now, and in another sense I am getting more comfortable talking about Ann in an objective, uninvolved way. I can say things like 'My wife died in June' without feeling a wrench inside. I can almost use the word 'widower' about myself. I began to come into the seminary in the morning more, because I don't need to be on transfer duty at home, and I go looking for coffee in the office. An assistant asked me if there were days I would like her to make sure the coffee was made. I explained that I had no actual routine; I was still finding my way into a routine after Ann died; and I could say that fairly dispassionately.

Ann's birthday came in the middle of the month. (She shared her birthday with Prince Charles; her family used to joke that the reason the BBC played the national anthem that day was to celebrate her birthday.) A friend emailed because she had seen from her calendar that it was Ann's birthday and she had guessed it would be one of those hard occasions. 'I remember celebrating her birthday once. You made a meal with mushrooms because she loved mushrooms. We listened to the Beatles, especially songs featuring John Lennon because she fancied him. It was a great celebration of a wonderful life.' It reminded me of her enthusiasm for the man I used to call the other love of her life, Simon Rattle, then the conductor of the City of Birmingham Symphony Orchestra.

The conference at New Orleans again meant meeting people I had not seen since she died. Some knew about it; some didn't. It was another, concentrated time of having the fact of her death being brought home. It is a little as if their shock and sadness at the news, or their need to register their sadness if they did already know, took me back to my initial shock and sadness and makes me experience it again. That is okay; I am inclined to want to cry each time, and I do so if the conversation goes on, but I don't mind. I had a helpful conversation with a friend who lost his own wife to cancer twenty years ago just after she had a baby, and who had thus lived through a bereavement more horrible than mine. Even at that time we both knew that eventually this would likely happen to me, though we would have expected it to happen much sooner, and we both knew now that this was in the background of the conversation. I knew he knew something of what I felt, and he knew that I knew something of what he had felt. Even though for both of us there was something upsetting about this conversation (taking place in the middle of a publisher's book display), he pointed out that we would not be honouring Ann if we did not have it. He added that the sense of loss never goes away. (Oh, thanks.) In general, if I could adjust easily to being alone, that would not be honouring her. As I type that now, and weep, I realize afresh that this is why it is not only okay but good for me to have the upsetting conversations. Once more I honour Ann and honour her memory and honour what she meant to me.

The first evening I went down Bourbon Street with friends and had a great time. The second evening I went down Bourbon Street on my own and had a great time. I have been aware over the past five months that I like my own company. I loved being with Ann and never wanted to be on my own apart from her, but now that she is gone, I like just being on my own (I am less of an extrovert than I present).

Month Five came to an end with Thanksgiving. I had declined people's caring invitations to Thanksgiving because I never feel quite part of this cultural celebration and because we enjoyed going to Paradise Cove in Malibu and sitting on the beach on our own. It was a perfect day, sunny and warm, yet to me it felt just okay, and when I got home I felt not depressed but indifferent or morose, and not full of appreciation as I usually feel when I get home from the beach. We had no strong tradition of going to that particular beach; it's ten or fifteen minutes further than our usual destination, and not so wheelchair-friendly. I wondered if the beach in general was too much associated with Ann, if going there would join other things that I would no longer do; this seemed sad. One or two people wondered if Thanksgiving was a hard time to be alone; but not being from the United States, this doesn't seem to apply to me. Next day I was back to normal. I went to *Café 322* and danced with great energy. More likely this had been another week when circumstances had combined to open the wounds. I was also aware that the next day was the last day of month five and that each month has seemed as if it would be the end but has actually simply been a transition to something different. It's as if it is a wound that is healing but that has to be reopened every few weeks because there is still hurt inside that needs to be allowed to escape.

Month 6 (29 November – 28 December)

The next month there was another wedding. A woman in my class was due to marry another student on 2 January, but on the day after Thanksgiving in the ninth week of the quarter I received from her the kind of email that professors often receive at this stage of the quarter, to say that she didn't think she could meet the deadline for turning in papers. Except that in her case the reason was that she had just been told that she had a brain tumour. She was to have surgery in two weeks and in that connection they had brought forward their wedding to the following Saturday. (She later told me that they had been influenced by something I said in a lecture on Jeremiah, 'Entering into Christian marriage is one of the most magnificent statements of hope we can make in this world, topped only by bringing children into the world'—I think the latter part of the observation comes from Stanley Hauerwas.)

We prayed for her in the next and last class of the quarter. I now saw another aspect of my feelings about the earlier wedding. When I had looked down at this couple in their beauty and their pristine youthfulness, I now realized I had been fearful of the possibility that some gigantic boulder was going to fall on them and shatter them, a boulder of the kind that fell on Ann and me and has fallen on this more recent couple. I found myself wanting to repeat Tony's lines to Maria in *West Side Story* when he passionately longs to take her far, far away from the troubles that are massing around them. (Actually he is about to be shot.) I felt as if I wanted to take this couple into my arms and whisk them off from what life could do to them. I suppose I wished there had been a way Ann and I could have been whisked away like that or that I could have whisked Ann off. I remembered something from the time after one of Ann's earlier bouts of pneumonia. Our patio has a wooden arbour over the gateway leading into the common area of the apartment grounds. A wisteria grows on the arch, but in my imagination I could also see the sword of Damocles hanging from the top of the arch waiting to fall on us.

I commented to a friend that this more recent bride was such a young slip of a thing to be facing what she is facing, but the friend was herself about to have a biopsy, and she responded, 'Girls are made out of steel, it's a scam that we look so fragile.' I knew that was true of this woman, as it was of this bride, and as it had been of Ann. I realized that in a way my reaction had been odd because I know the boulder didn't shatter us even though the sword did eventually fall.

My colleague Erin Dufault-Hunter introduced the brought-forward marriage service with these words:

> There are at least two things I have decided to do that (it turns out) I had *no idea* what I was saying when I said I would do them: One was to follow Jesus, the other was to get married. All of us make commitments, make promises to care and love other people—to join our lives with others'—and yet we have no real idea what we are doing. When we gather for weddings, such uncertainties are often in the background, and the focus is on the couple and their love for one another, our shared hopes for their future. Sometimes we can indulge the illusion that it is our human love in the form of romance that sustains us and makes such promises possible. This wedding is different. Adrianne and Nathan do not have the luxury of pretending that they know what they are doing today, because they are acutely aware that they are not in control of their future. They do not know what the diagnosis will be or the nature of Adrianne's recovery. Adrianne and Nathan have no idea what they are promising when they link their lives together in their vows, and we have no idea what we are doing, when we promise by our presence here

at this Christian wedding to sustain, support, and protect this marriage as their community. But Christian marriage is not about what *we* know, nor about what *we* are able to do to keep our promises, nor about *our* ability to sustain ourselves or control our futures. Rather, Christian marriage is about the One who invites us to make such promises. It is a celebration of the God who by *his* faithfulness makes such crazy commitments possible—and, most importantly, infuses them with the deepest joy in the keeping of them. Nathan and Adrianne welcome you into their future, not because they are sure what it entails, but because they trust in the One who transforms foolish promises to love another into the wisdom that nourishes an abundant life.

I sat in a pew crying. (The next Thursday the surgeons couldn't find the tumour they had been convinced was there.)

This was also the month I began to feel lonely, which was a surprise; but each month has been a surprise in a different way. Immediately after Ann died I wanted to be alone. I didn't want people coming to bring me food or offer me condolences or take me out. I wanted to be alone to process what had happened. I have noted that I also thought that being alone might be my natural style. People who know me would laugh, because I present as a party-loving person, but I suspect there is something misleading there. When I was a child, at extended family parties I remember sitting behind the sofa reading a book. When Ann and I studied counseling according to the Frank Lake system, I came out as schizoid. On at least one occasion when I have done Myers-Briggs, I have come out as introvert. I used to joke that introverts are people who want to hide, and I hide by pretending to be extrovert; I am not sure whether it was just a joke. I don't like parties or other such occasions where I don't know people and I have to make my way in strange company. I was reverting to an aspect of my natural style.

Subsequent to that initial desire to be alone, I was troubled by the fact that the house was empty, but I didn't mean I was troubled because no one was there; I was troubled because Ann wasn't there, it was empty of her. I now had a different sense of aloneness. The same week my sleeping pattern went odd again, almost as odd as it was for weeks three and four though not actually as wearing. I would go to sleep okay then wake up after a couple of hours and stay awake for an hour, then sleep again for another four. This was the point at which I thought maybe I should see a therapist, but as usual, when I had articulated all this, it felt as if the problem might be solved. I had to adjust to being on my own. Perhaps I could do that.

I spent Christmas in England with my sons and their families. I loved being with them, and it was especially apt that (by coincidence) we were all together for dinner on 28 December, the sixth-month anniversary of Ann's death. I did not really feel that it being the first Christmas without Ann made the celebration difficult, which is what you are supposed to feel; maybe this is because I am not much of a 'special occasion' person anyway. I enthuse about celebrating the Jesus story but as a social occasion Christmas doesn't mean much more to me than Thanksgiving. We had some good conversations about Ann, which usually upset me somewhat, but that was okay. I loved seeing England again and rediscovering how lovely it is, and I imagined being happy about going back to live there if I had to. I saw my sister and her husband, and we joked about me living in an apartment across the street from the quay and beach at St Ives in Cornwall, where decades ago I had romanced about Ann and me living in retirement, with me shuffling across the street with my walking frame to sit on the bench above the beach. We talked slightly more seriously about the idea of my going to live with her and her husband one day. But I was ready to come back to Los Angeles, anticipating the moment when the pilot says 'We are about to begin our descent to LA, where it is a warm and clear evening and the temperature is seventy degrees.'

Month 7 (29 December – 28 January)

While I allowed for the theoretical possibility that the New Year might bring something new, I did not expect it to do so, and once again I was mistaken. It related to that sense of the down side to being alone. I have noted a colleague's comment that 'my experience as a pastor does not lead me to romanticize such circumstances' as the ones Ann and I had lived with. Since her illness took its turn for the worse nearly thirty years ago I have missed there being someone who could give herself unequivocally to me and to whom I could give myself unequivocally. In this respect I have been like some single people I know who long that there should be someone with whom they have that mutual commitment, though I have been even more like some married people who lack that reality even though they are married.

In the past, in my imagination I have turned several individuals into that person. I have spoiled at least one friendship by doing so, though more often the fantasizing goes on only inside my head, and (as far as I am aware) the other person doesn't know about it. Everyone has thought I was committed to Ann heart and soul, and they are not exactly wrong. I have committed my life to her, but I have not exactly succeeded in committing my imagination. In addition, while I have not committed adultery in the full sense, I have had relationships that I should not have had, with varying degrees of physical intimacy. I guess I craved for a living relationship with someone of the kind Ann and I once had. It was two decades before I got some handle on the dynamics of all this.

I have mentioned that when Ann died, we had tickets for eight concerts over the summer, and I sent emails around people we knew to see if they would like to come in this dead person's place. I thus found myself taking women as well as men to the concerts, and when the tickets ran out, I invited some of these women as well as men, and some others, to go to other concerts. When I went with a woman, these weren't dates. Admittedly, I'm not absolutely sure what a date is. One of them told me she had been on a date so I asked how she knew it was a date, and she told me it came about through a dating service, so that both helped and didn't help. On these non-dates, I didn't necessarily pay for both of us, the evenings didn't imply that this might be the beginning of something much more serious and more exclusive, and I was pretty sure that the women didn't view them that way. To start with, while some of the women were near my own age, most were students or recent graduates, typically people in their thirties ('and you get paid to do this job as well?' a friend commented). They had all known Ann or knew I had just lost her. They were not people who (as far as I know) would imagine themselves hooked up with a man so much older than them; the relationships were not equal or plausible ones. Yet this did not stop me fantasizing about the possible greater significance of these relationships. If all these women had other things to do than hang out with me, this hurt me. (Gee, I hope none of them ever reads this.)

One particular week I asked about four of them out, and none could come (it was the week before Christmas, and they all had good reason to be busy). A good thing about that fourfold 'No' was that it reminded me not to fantasize. It reminded me that the other people were not fantasizing about me in the way I was about them. My position now Ann has died is even more like that of a single person.

Most of the people who were not free to go out with me have no family community here in California but have developed alternative 'families'; they have friends and communities of some kind. I had such a community in Nottingham, but it disappeared when we moved. I had another community in California for a while, but it dissolved through people moving away. My fantasizing issued in part from having no such community and focussing everything on the idea of one person. Maybe I also need a community, and need to put my energy into developing a community rather than into spending time with one person, though you can't manufacture a community. At least, I didn't make my previous communities happen. They simply happened.

To articulate much of this awareness is to articulate the novelty of the New Year. I realized what I had been doing in seeking a kind of substitute for Ann and realized that I not only should but could grow out of doing it. I could not have seen things this way a month or two previously. From time to time over the six months since Ann died people have expressed the hope that I might find new joys or new experiences or something along those lines, and they naturally did this on Christmas cards and in New Year greetings, but I wasn't always sure what they meant. While the wish may be as open as it sounds, I suspected that some were expressing the hope that I would find a new relationship, or that they were encouraging me to do so. One or two half-implied the hope that it would involve less of the grief of the old relationship (though I myself don't really see the old one as centrally characterized by grief).

People say you should wait a year after losing someone before making any big decisions, and this would include developing relationships. I had been thinking I would wait a year before even thinking about the question, but sometimes it seemed as if the question was pressing itself on me. I had thought I could not imagine reorganizing my life around someone else, having been for two or three decades perforce in control of the relationship I had with Ann, and of our life together. But perhaps I could relish having to do that reorganizing. It would be an aspect of the newness. For some reason, I also began to feel easier about facing Ann on resurrection day if I should marry someone else. I happened to be reading 1 Corinthians, and I imagined myself waiting eagerly for the appearing of Jesus (1 Corinthians 1:7) when I will be able to hold hands with Ann and with other people I have come to love.

As the month wore on I twisted and turned about these questions. Sometimes I was happy with my way of managing a number of friendships. Sometimes I felt especially attracted to one person. Sometimes I thought someone might be interested in me; sometimes I didn't think any of the people I knew would be. I examined tiny details in their reactions to me. What did that hug mean? What did those sign-off words at the end of an email mean? I reflected that I was like any single person in fretting over these questions. I wondered whether I would settle into acceptance of my singleness. And I was doing all this as a guy aged 67, for goodness sake!

I watched the movie *(500) Days of Summer*, about the relationship between two people that is premised on his being in love with her and thinking she is in love with him, when actually she is uncertain of her feelings for him. He thus gets desperately hurt. I could identify with both the man and the woman. I could give the impression that I am interested in someone when I am not. Or I could think they are interested in me when they are not. A hug or a greeting may easily be simply expressions of friendship love, but might indicate an openness to romantic love. What did I want them to mean? It's much easier for a woman (under the old rules). You just have to wait for a man to take the initiative.

There were other new features of this seventh month. Each Wednesday in seminary chapel I had wanted to sit where I always sat with Ann. This is odd in a way, because there are many places I have not wanted to go to because we used to go there, and these include our own patio as well as clubs. Whatever the reason for the difference, in the first chapel of the New Year I knew it was time to sit somewhere else, somewhere in the main body of the auditorium. It would signify being my own person, it would acknowledge that there was no need to sit where we used to sit because the wheelchair fitted there, and it would signify that it is a new year, a new stage in my life.

And I went with a friend for the free swing dancing lesson that precedes the dance itself. I am extremely incompetent and will never get it. But I had great fun.

Month 8 (29 January – 28 February)

On the last day of January I went to see the Rodgers and Hammerstein musical *Carousel*. I knew it would make me cry, and it did, though I didn't realize I would start crying in the overture and do so intermittently all the way through, at more than one point fearing that people on either side would be aware of my shaking as I tried to restrain this weeping. Afterwards as I walked back to the parking lot among hundreds of middle-aged and older couples arm in arm or hand in hand, I wanted to seize them by the shoulders and say DON'T TAKE FOR GRANTED THAT YOU ARE LIKE THAT.

The *New York Times* has a weekly page called 'Modern Love' in which each week someone recounts an experience of a relationship (not necessarily romantic—sometimes they are about (say) parenthood or dogs). On Valentine's Day the page's editor reflected on some of the stories and commented on some of the issues they raise, such as whether it is acceptable to dump someone by email message and (more significantly for me) what happens when two people are friends but one of them 'suddenly wants more', starts falling in love, 'exhibits a slight change in body language, or a misinterpreted glance or smile'? Then 'the equilibrium shifts irreparably' and the friendship collapses. The editor's 'solution' sounds easy. You just squash it and forget it. You knew the basis of the relationship. Deal with it.

In my reading of 1 Corinthians I reached chapter 7, which encourages people who have been widowed to stay single if they have the gift. I guess I have the gift; in some key ways I have been living like a single person for years. Anne Roiphe closes her memoir about bereavement, *Epilogue*, by concluding that she will likely never again have a soul mate and that she will miss sex, and miss someone to share things with, but that she will be okay. I can imagine that working; I have enough good friends to share things with so as to be able to manage without a 'dedicated' soul mate, even if I never have a community. I am again like any other single person for whom there isn't someone with whom I have an exclusive mutual commitment but who can get by if there are people with whom there is a degree of mutual commitment. If I spread myself around, maybe there is blessing for others too, as there used to be when Ann was alive. A good chunk of me hates that idea of making a commitment to singleness, but it would be typical if that was what God wanted. I said to God, 'That's tough. But it's typical of you to be tough. I tell people you are tough. It's partly because you are a trainer. And it's okay. I know that works.' God said, 'Yes.' I reflected, 'But it was easy when the training was in effect imposed on me. It's harder when I have to choose it.' And God said, 'That's the next stage of training.'

Maybe I don't need to commit myself to that stance forever but simply to take it as a *modus vivendi*, a decision until something else happens, such as that I fall for someone or someone asks me for a date. If I think in those terms, I can be more relaxed about the friends I have and not be anxious (one of Paul's concerns in 1 Corinthians 7). This question was not one that got resolved by the end of Month Eight. Indeed, I was no further on with it, but the processing was important. Perhaps it's not the kind of question that gets resolved, unless I do actually make a commitment to someone or make an actual vow to stay single.

Years ago, Ann introduced me to the work of Colin Murray Parkes, a British psychiatrist whom she once knew slightly in London and who is the great British guru on bereavement. One of his insights is that after someone dies we may spend much time and energy trying to find the person again. I can see the way I had been doing this in yearning for a relationship with someone. A friend of mine who has said she can never imagine marrying again says (in effect) that this is so because she can never imagine finding her husband again, and he is the person she wants. For me the dynamics include a converse element, that there was so much that Ann could not be for me for most of the time of our marriage and I yearn for the kind of relationship we had in the earlier years. I am trying to find Ann as she was in the 1970s.

This month, I was ready to dispose of Ann's clothes. I had speculated a few months ago that the New Year was the time I would do this, and it now feels right. On the other hand, I gave up going to Malibu for lunch from time to time, the way we used to together. It seems aimless now she is not with me. Sitting alone for lunch isn't the same. Instead I put my bike in the car that fortuitously has room for it, because the back seat folds, and I went to Venice Beach, and rode along the boardwalk for three or four miles to Pacific Palisades, stopping once or twice to eat a sandwich or look at the view. I decided to experiment, go to different beaches and try out different restaurants. On Valentine's Day I went to the beach, parked in a lot I had never used before and rode along a stretch of the boardwalk where I had not previously been. (I didn't worry about the fact that my front brake had snapped the previous night, but in those circumstances I was a bit more careful than usual among the bikers and walkers and roller-bladers; it was a beautiful day and Los Angeles was out at the beach in force.) I bought chicken quesadilla at a beach café where I had not previously eaten and sat on a beach I had not previously visited. I slept on the sand where I had not previously slept and read a new book.

Month 9   (1–28 March)

As usual I didn't expect anything new in this new month but at the end of the first week I discerned something. This time it was not something painful. I thought I had stopped looking for someone who would replace Ann. Maybe this exactly proves the wisdom that says 'Don't get involved with someone for a year in case you are simply on the rebound.' I wondered whether maybe, just maybe, I had stopped fantasizing. When Ann was alive, and then after she died, I wanted to fill in the hole that was caused by her illness and then by her death. Maybe, just maybe, the hole had filled itself in, like the hole of a wound healing, and I didn't have to look for someone to fill it. Maybe if I do find that I want to commit myself to someone, there is more chance that I will want to commit myself to that person in her own right.

A contractor came to fix a problem with the electrics in our apartment. He remembered that Ann had been there on a previous occasion and he told me about his own divorce a couple of years ago. He talked about his loneliness, though he also commented on the fact that there are lots of unattached women around, and I was not clear why he was avoiding getting involved. When I said I was okay about being on my own he expressed astonishment. On another day I was talking to a friend whose father had died some years ago. His parents' marriage had not been happy and he described his mother as longing to marry again, hoping that all the pain of that first marriage could be replaced by a happy marital experience. I realized that in my own way this is what I had been doing, but I thought that maybe now I had stopped doing it. I still thought that it would be great to make love to someone at night and great to wake up in the morning with that person, though I'm still not so sure about the other sixteen hours of the day. Marriage involves reshaping your life around or with this other person. There is a sense in which from a selfish viewpoint I am better off forgoing that positive aspect of marriage in order to keep my life the way it is. It also means I get more writing done (what a pathetic piece of logic!). And it avoids the prospect of my becoming a burden to someone as I grow frailer.

Freud suggested (I read somewhere) that mourners need to reclaim energy that they had expended on the loved one they had lost. Any relationship uses energy; I suppose that my relationship with Ann may have used more energy than most people's relationship with the one they love. Paradoxically, mourning, which seems like a purely negative experience of loss, is a kind of regrouping and reframing. The notion of regrouping usually presupposes a negative experience, an experience of defeat. There is a sense in which Ann's death represented a victory rather than a defeat. I had looked after her as best I could and made it possible for her to fulfil her ministry, and eventually she and God had decided that enough was enough, and I had been dismissed, or we had both been dismissed. She was free to rest and I was free to start over. In that sense it is a positive regrouping, a new start. It thus also is a reframing of yourself and your life. I know what I used to be about; I can now be about something different. I don't know what that will be, though this is probably because I am never very good at deciding what to be or do so that I can then go for it; I am inclined just to let life happen to me. This is not very American, but I am happy with where it has got me in life. It's not much like Paul or David (or Jesus?) but it's quite like Abraham or Moses (or God?). So I will find out what the new John Goldingay will be by noting what happens. I no longer feel that my life is over, that I am just treading water until I die. I have so many classes to teach and so many books to write and so many relationships to encourage and so much music to enjoy.

I used to belong to the *When Harry Met Sally* school with regard to relationships with women; I believed that friendships with women are impossible because sex always gets in the way. I think I have got most of the way out of that. I now have friendships with women that indeed derive their fun partly from my being a man and the other person being a woman, so that sex does feature. But it's not as if the time you spend together is really foreplay, so that it fails to reach its natural end because you don't end up in bed. (Another definition of a date, or of what is not a date, according to an episode of *The West Wing*, which I have been re-watching: 'It won't be a date, because there will be no sex at the end of the evening.') That also means I have a community; it's just that it doesn't all meet together.

On the last Saturday of the nine months, the day before the actual nine months anniversary, I went to the beach on my own again. It was another beautiful day and Los Angeles was out at the beach in force again. I rode to the pier, walked the length of it and had strawberry daiquiri and beef fajitas in the sunshine at the last Mexican restaurant before you reach New Zealand. I thought about riding the Ferris Wheel (I have never done that), but there was a long line; maybe I will do it next time. I rode back to the parking lot and lay in the sand to sleep. I came home and sat on the patio for the rest of the day. I had not sat there like that since Ann died, because when she was alive we spent so much time there. But now I have reclaimed it.

I thought, 'I can do this, this life without Ann, this new life.'

ACKNOWLEDGMENTS

For comments that appear in this book or otherwise shaped it, I am grateful to family, friends, colleagues, and students in England and in California, specifically to Adrianne and Nathan Penner, Alec Motyer, Amy Drennan, Amy Meverden, Andrea Haller, Anne Long, Antony Miller, Bill Goodman, Brian Lugioyo, Cathy Schaller, Charles Read, Chris Wright, Christine and Alldrin Penamora, Clifton Clarke, Colin Buchanan, Colin Moody, David Monteith, Dottie and Fred Davison, Doug McConnell, Elaine Labourel, Ellen Charry, Erika Carney Haub, Erin Dufault-Hunter, Ernesto Tinajero, Francis Bridger, Graham and Molly Dow, Gene Rogers, Gerald Janzen, Grayson Carter (whose idea this book was), Hazel Michelson, Jeremy Trew, Jill Murphy, Lesley Evans, Lisa Lee Miller, Marianne Meye Thompson, Mark Goldingay, Mark Labberton, Matt Lumpkin, Mike Lotzer, Morag Fowler, Pieter and Elria Kwant, Richard Turner, Roger Finney, Scilla Yates, Sheila Whitmore, Sol Nuñez, Steve Mann, Steven Goldingay, Sue and Phil Groom, Tanner Searles, Tom Parker, Tom Smail, Úna Lucey-Lee, and Walter Moberly.

I have adapted a few sentences from *The Usual Suspects* (Carlisle: Paternoster, 1998), which appeared in a US edition as *Walk On* (Grand Rapids: Baker, 2002). It is out of print but the text appears at http://campusguides.fuller.edu/johngoldingay . It gives more detail on various aspects of Ann's story.   *John Goldingay*

Afterword

Just after returning to the publisher the edited version of this book, I read an account of criticisms concerning a similar memoir that had not mentioned how the author had remarried thirteen months after her husband's death. The English novelist Julian Barnes had commented that she had breached the principle of narrative promise.

A few months after submitting the original manuscript, I met Kathleen Scott and (as the back cover notes) we have since married. A story that seemed to have come to an end for me, suddenly became a story that was unfinished.

I could write a further chapter to this book about romancing and getting married again in my late sixties. Yet that would compromise the point about this book as I wrote it, which was to honour Ann in light of how significant a person she was to me and to other people, and to reflect on the process of losing her.

For me, it was important to reach the point where this book ends, with my gaining the confidence to say 'I can do this, this life without Ann, this new life.' With hindsight, I see how important it was to reach that point before I could properly or safely fall in love with somebody else. But reaching that point actually is the ending of a story. Meeting Kathleen is the beginning of different one.

John Goldingay

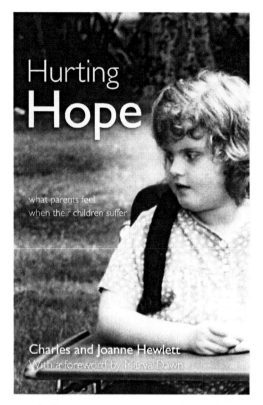

HURTING HOPE
what parents feel when their children suffer

by Charles and Joanne Hewlett

ISBN 9781903689745

www.piquanteditions.com

CPSIA information can be obtained at www.ICGtesting.com
Printed in the USA
268454BV00006B/2/P